MW01624469

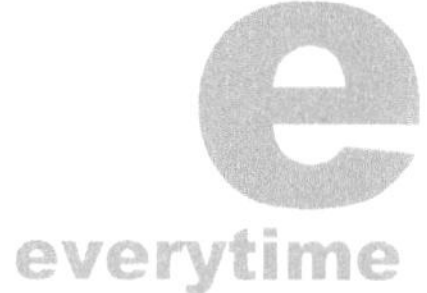
e
everytime

DAMN THE PONYTAIL

MATT DEVIRGILIIS

First published November 2021

BP#00109

Everytime Press
32 Meredith Street
Sefton Park SA 5083
Australia

Email: edpureslush@live.com.au
Website: https://pureslush.com/
Store: https://pureslush.com/store/

ISBN: 978-1-922427-72-4

Also available as ePub and Kindle eBooks
ePub ISBN: 978-1-922427-80-9
Kindle ISBN: 978-1-922427-96-0

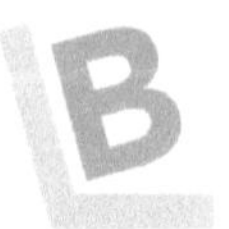

Everytime Press is a member of the
Bequem Publishing collective
https://bequempublishing.com/

DEDICATED TO

THE DADS

We sat next to the incubator – a slow cooker for babies – watching our three-pound daughter lie as if she were a gecko in the zoo's reptile house. My wife and I were already through our first week of this type of parenting. And lucky for us – if you'd call it that – we knew ahead of time that we'd be in this situation. We'd been given a tour of the NICU, met the nurses and doctors, and learned about the various monitors. A week in and it felt nearly normal. We knew nothing different.

In walked a S.W.A.T. team of nurses pushing a newborn and performing their miracles. A father stood on his tiptoes behind them, his hands clasped behind his head. He wore no religious symbols and said nothing aloud, but his face split between horror and prayer. He wasn't as lucky. No tour. No prep. His wife went into labor. It was supposed to be happy. But they wound up in the NICU.

In sitting down to write this, I realized that no one would care about my story. My girls and wife maybe. They can read this to understand what went through my head as their births unfolded. But at that moment, seeing that new dad's sad and confused face, I realized that fathers have very little prep. Sure there are books pretending to have the secret ten steps to parenting. They're garbage. I always tell people the only guaranteed parental advice anyone can give is to ignore the parental advice you get. You figure it out as you go.

This book isn't about advice. It's to let the dads out there know that you are not alone. If you can relate to just one story or if one of these situations makes you laugh, then I've accomplished my goal.

AND TO

THE NURSES AND DOCTORS

Every parent who steps into the NICU is terrified. Even if parents get a tour beforehand, they are still scared to all hell. The doctors and nurses who dedicate their time to the babies, parents, and families are saints. There's no other way to describe them. Thank you for keeping my girls alive.

AND TO

MY BABER

Brittany, my wife, is the nucleus of our family. Every day I'm impressed by just how selfless a wife and mom she is. I wouldn't have been able to write this if it weren't for her … and not just because it's the story of us and our daughters, but because she gave me the time and the space to craft and to toil.

As prolific a writer as I may be, I still find it difficult to put down to paper how much I love her. So for now –

Thank you, Brittany, my Baber. I love you.

CONTENTS

LIL BEAR

1 Land, Wash, Takeoff, Land, Drive
4 Phone Calls to Loved Ones
6 How We Got Here
8 Virtual Throat Punch
11 How the Hell Do You Spell Preemie
13 Hospital Room Easter Dinner
15 First Lie
17 Outside the O.R.
19 4:15
22 Welcome to the N.I.C.U.
24 Afterbirth
26 Earth Angels
30 That's a Diaper
31 Sibling Visits
34 Unfiltered Nurse
38 Going Home Alone
41 Holding You (Kangaroo)
44 Settle Down, Settle Down
46 The Songs We Sing
48 First Bottle

50 One Month
53 Passing Tests
56 Going Home Together
58 Not a Doll
61 Lil Shit

LAINEY KATE

67 A Pistol From the Start
68 Whatta?
71 Phone Calls to Family … Again
73 Loving Two
75 Choice
77 Goddamn Ponytails
79 Shower Cry
81 Hemorrhage
84 I Don't Want to Die
86 She's a Whopper
89 I'm an Anesiesiologist
91 Count 'Em
92 We Got This N.I.C.U. Thing
94 Parents to the Respite
96 2am Code Red
99 Tiny Slice

100 Five-Day Wait
103 Brittany's Scar
105 Who Needs Skin?
107 Empty Handed Again
108 The Songs We Sing
110 Sibling Visits
111 Dirty Peter Rabbit
113 Lil Meet Lainey
115 Late-Night Stops as the Inlet
117 Don't Argue Statistical Significance with Me
121 Christmas Breakfast with Santa
124 Home
125 Afterthoughts

127 About the Author

128 Thanks

LIL BEAR

LAND, WASH, TAKEOFF, LAND, DRIVE

"You have to come home. Now. And by home, I mean the hospital. The doctors said I can't leave."

My taxi carves through morning Minneapolis rush hour traffic on 35W while I ping-pong in the backseat.

Brittany speaks through the phone.

Tears pour down my cheeks.

It's colder than hell in February. No sign of spring. I wipe my scarf across my face to dry the moisture so it doesn't freeze outside.

She's 28-weeks pregnant. I don't expect to hear these words come from her mouth. But these are the words she says and the words I hear.

She's in New Jersey and I'm in Minnesota.

My life as a consultant has put me on the road every week for nearly a year, flying from home in the garden state to Minneapolis every Monday morning and flying back every Thursday night.

"I'm okay," she says, "and the baby is okay. They just have to do everything possible to keep her cooking. And you just have to get home as soon as you can. Don't be scared, though. And my mom is on her way."

"Thank god," I say. My mother-in-law is one of the main reasons I've continued the road-warrior with such ease. She lives around the corner and provides support all of the time. There've been many a punchline about mothers-in-law. My own breaks every stereotype. She's selfless. She's strong. And her being with Brittany is the best comfort I can hear. "I'm so glad she'll be there with you," I say. She hangs up to call other doctors and leaves me to my own imagination.

I'm not scared. Just going to pass out in the backseat of this decrepit cab, but I can blame the heavy scent of body odor.

We pull into the hotel driveway and someone opens the door. "Good morning, Mr. D.," says Andrew. "You're here early." He grabs my arm as I stagger out of the car and test my legs. "Everything okay?" he asks.

"I have to get back to the airport. Fast. Brittany is in labor but it's way too soon."

"Come in and wash up first. Your room is ready. Bring some color back to your face. D will drive you back to the airport."

Carla behind the counter hands me a keycard. "Heard what you said," she says. "Use the room. We'll remove your reservation after you leave."

The employees here are like family, having put up with me every week for almost a year. We're on a first-name basis. They know what's going on in my life and I in theirs. Even D the driver knows me. His name is long and hard to pronounce so everyone just calls him D. Only the letter D is on his business cards and only the letter D is saved in my phone.

I also like to think that they like me because I'm not a whiny traveler who thinks status makes me a snowflake. I have no special requests. Just hope to have a room early in the morning so I can scrub the airplane germs from my skin. Now they're taking care of me like family.

The elevator moves slowly, as if checking on each floor as we pass by. It will take years to get to the 15th floor.

After a five-minute shower, I bolt downstairs, dart through the lobby, thank my hotel family – hugs included – and jump in the car. D and I careen back to the airport.

PHONE CALLS TO LOVED ONES

"Hi. Brittany's in labor," I say to my mom. Details, details, details. Sobbing.

"She'll be okay," she says, "and call Dad."

"Hi. Brittany's in labor," I say to my dad. Details, details, details. Sobbing.

"She'll be okay," he says, "and call your siblings."

"Hi. Brittany's in labor." Sobbing.

"Hi. Brittany's in labor." Sobbing.

The calls get easier, like watching myself deliver the same lines in a movie over and over again. But the reality sets in – my wife is in labor way too early. The next few weeks are up in the air. Our baby will be premature. And I'm still hours away from being able to hug Brittany.

D punches the gas in his Jaguar and we speed down the highway back to the airport. "Maybe you should put the phone down for a minute," he says.

I do. Opening my window, the cold air smacks my face and fills the car. The sun sits just above the treeline. I notice a brown and white hawk perched on a bare branch, breast feathers puffed up.

We're close to the airport.

"Thanks and bye," I say and sprint from D's car.

"Good luck," he says as the sliding doors shut.

"Thanks," I say again through the glass.

Lines are short. "You can fly standby on a flight that boards in 30 minutes," says the ticketing agent. She hands me a paper ticket and hands me back my driver's license. "Have a good flight."

The back of the plane is full. A church group piles in and pins me against the window. They wear the same red shirts and chatter with identical pep in their voices. I'd like to hit them but their cheer picks me up. Since I was a kid, car rides and plane rides put me to sleep. Give me five minutes on a 737 and I'm out like a hibernating bear. Not this time. There's too much on my mind. The plane pushes off and the pilot provides our planned altitude. And I pass out. An hour later, I wake to the same lively Christian clamor. How could I fall to sleep when my world is in such turmoil? I'm so sorry. Guilt streams through my veins. Throwing a few punches would be therapeutic. I say a few Our Fathers instead.

HOW WE GOT HERE

"Are you okay?" I knock on the closed bathroom door. Brittany's third time in a few minutes. She comes out of the bathroom and rummages through the linen closet and squats to avoid bending over with her beautiful, pregnant belly.

"I guess I'm going to be one of those women who pee themselves toward the end of their pregnancy," she says. "Figures. We haven't gone through enough already."

She is gorgeous. Pregnant. Gorgeous. Stressed. Gorgeous. "What's wrong?" I ask.

"I'm leaking. Figure the baby is bouncing on my bladder. Doesn't smell like pee though." She smiles. "Don't worry. I called the doctor and left a message with the answering service. They said the doctor should call back."

"Do you still want to go?"

"I guess so." Her smile hides her underlying fear. She's not much for exploring the unknown and right now her leaking is an unknown. No matter how much she researches online, she will stress until the doctor calls. She'd prefer to stay safe and home.

We planned to head into New York City. Grab lunch at New York Beer Company and see *Matilda* in previews. "We don't have to," I say.

"I'm just peeing myself like a little kid. And it's not much," she says. "We shouldn't skip a fun day for that."

So we get ready, pushing the unknown out of the way. Brittany stands in front of her long mirror, tilting her head to the left as she examines how the clothes flow along her curves. We jump in the car, jump on the train, devour pretzels, and down fried chicken sandwiches. Then we marvel at the talented kids in the play. Four hours later, we reverse course and head home. No calls from the doctor.

I take off for Minneapolis the next morning. Her doctor calls while I'm mid-flight. Turns out we should have been worried. Brittany is leaking uterine fluid. Not just pee. It's something to worry about, something concerning.

We didn't know and she was right – we enjoyed the night and left the stress behind.

She calls. "You have to come home."

I'm glad we got that night together.

VIRTUAL THROAT PUNCH

I'm a non-violent man. Sure, I've been in my share of grade school and high school fistfights. But never the aggressor. I stay calm until a line is crossed. And I do all I can to make sure that line is far away. I'm peaceful.

I sit in a waiting area at the end of one of the hospital hallways. Two chairs face each other and a TV hangs overhead, airing daytime soaps.

I just learned that Brittany was in labor and that even though she called the answering service that answering service never called the doctor. The answering service has one job – answer the phone when patients call, call the doctor, then call patients back. This service forgot the second and third steps. We're lucky Brittany's water didn't fully break on Broadway.

I'm pissed.

Because Brittany called as soon as I landed at the Minneapolis airport, I only thought about getting home as fast as possible. I didn't have time to call my bosses or my team. So I pick up the phone and call one of our leads – we'll call him Timmy.

"Timmy," I say, "It's Matt." I tell him the story. I fight back tears and take a breath. He says nothing for a minute, and I assume he's processing it and trying to find words to ease my worry.

"Who gave you permission to take days off?"

"What?"

"We have an important deadline. Who said you didn't have to be in Minneapolis and that you could go home?"

I'm a peaceful man. Never the aggressor. I pull the phone away from my ear and stare at it and think *what the fuck?*

"I'm sorry, Tim, what?"

"You heard me. Who gave you permission to go home?"

I'm a peaceful man. I quickly power-rank all the assholes I'd ever become angry with and realize Tim ranks number one. I want to reach through the phone and throat-punch the guy. Sure, he's my boss, but he can also go fuck himself. My blood courses hot and my nerves start to shake. My inner rage is about to erupt.

"Okay, Tim," I somehow say calmly into the phone. I cruise past the anger and say again, "Okay, Tim. I'll call you back." And I hang up on the asshole.

I call my other manager, Ed, and tell him the story. I tell him about Brittany and I tell him about Tim's response. It helps that this manager is also one of my best friends. "Do not worry about work," he says. "And I will handle Tim." I thank Ed and we hang up.

After a few minutes of deep breathing, I walk back to Brittany's hospital room. "Everything okay?" she asks.

"Everything is good," I say, "and Tim is an asshole."

HOW THE HELL DO YOU SPELL PREEMIE?

After sitting in the hospital for a few days Brittany and I realize it's for the best if I'm not around every second. Work distracts me. Brittany says she's feeling fine. Plus, I want to take time off when Liliana is born.

"You should go back to work," says Brittany. "Go and travel until it's actually time. I'll be fine and I'll tell you if I'm not."

It pains me to agree with her. I should be here for her. I should be chivalrous. I should jump when she needs. But she is tired of me taking work calls in her room. She doesn't need me sitting by her side and announcing her vitals. And I need the distraction from fear. So I agree.

At this point, everyone I work with knows what's going on. But every conversation begins and ends with, "Well, I'll have to see because my wife could go into labor at any minute." My client wants to schedule a working session … "Well, I'll have to see." They set a deadline. "I'll have to see."

Brittany is tired of hearing me type emails. The emails are the same. They all contain the same last paragraph – *Because my daughter will be a preemie – Because my daughter will be a premee – Because my daughter will be a premie –* .

"Baber?" I ask Brittany.

"Yeah?"

"How the hell do you spell preemie?"

"Use a double-e in the beginning," says Brittany. "It will be spelled that way on all of her clothes."

I finish my emails.

30-minutes later I'm writing another email and I get to the last paragraph – *Because my daughter will be a preemie – Because my daughter will be a premee – Because my daughter will be a premie –*.

"Baber?" I ask Brittany. "How the hell do you spell preemie?"

HOSPITAL ROOM EASTER DINNER

My mother-in-law hands out plates. Real plates. Glass or porcelain or whatever makes them shatter. She lays various sized containers across the hospital windowsill in front of the flowers and cards. The smells of turkey and sweet mashed potatoes fill the room. Brittany's family stands around, sits if they can. Brittany has her own room complete with two beds.

We pile food onto our plates. We chatter, shoveling sides into our mouths between potshots and laughs. Nurses come in, take vitals, fill their own dishes, then leave.

Normal Easter dinner in an abnormal location. We enjoy ourselves and I eat too much.

"How is it?" asks Brittany's mom. I'm loading up on my second helping.

"It's okay, Mom," says Brittany. "It's okay."

We stack the plates and scrape the food bits into the hospital room's tall trashcan. Brittany's mom closes the lids on the food containers and stacks them in a carrying bag. "We'll go now," she says. We chatter for a while longer, joking and laughing. Her family hugs and kiss us, hugging Brittany harder.

They leave. The room is quiet except for the fetal heart monitor's beeping. Brittany falls to sleep in her bed. I sit on the opposite bed and write a letter to my en route daughter. The room darkens. My eyes close and my many thoughts slide into my dreams.

FIRST LIE

Brittany grabs her stomach. She's doubled over in bed.

Running in, I ask for details. "What's going on? What's the doctor saying?"

"I'm just glad you made it home so fast," says Brittany. She winces as she talks to me. "Doctor says that he'll wait as long as he can but no promises. If he needs to deliver, he'll do it without you."

I reach out and take her hand. As we clasp one another she bites her lower lip and squeezes my fingers until they're almost purple.

"I'm having contractions and have a fever. That's why I asked you to come home. Had a feeling."

"Contractions?"

"The baby wants out. At least we made it to thirty weeks."

Brittany's mom sits on a pink chair beside the bed. "Doctor said they'll bring her in as soon as you get here."

A nurse pops in. "Okay, Brittany, the doctor is ready in the OR. We'll wheel you over. Do you think you can get out of bed and sit on the wheelchair on your own?"

"I think so," says Brittany. One hand on her stomach, she lurches forward. I guide her and she grimaces. "God it hurts so bad. Feels like I'm bleeding a lot." Brittany slowly walks a few steps and leans back into the wheelchair. The nurse spins her around toward the door. "Am I bleeding?" she asks.

Her mom and I peek at the hospital bed. It looks like a lion mauled an antelope.

"Nothing," I say.

This is the only lie I've ever told her.

OUTSIDE THE O.R.

The hall is empty and glows green. Clinks and clanks echo through the large OR door. Brittany is behind the door, surrounded by a horde of bustling doctors and nurses. All this effort to deliver our very early baby Lil. My breaths speed up. Small sections of my mask pop in and out like ground swelling before a volcanic eruption. My paper scrubs envelop my body, somehow baggy and strangling. The hall lengthens.

"She'll be okay," says a man in scrubs as he leaves the OR. "Don't worry." He pats my shoulder. "You can sit next to her in a minute." He disappears back into the room. Through the closing door, I see Brittany, a cap over her hair and her head tilted toward me, splayed out on the table like naked Jesus.

The door snaps shut. The hall grows longer and the clanking grows more distant. My cries behind this mask are silent. Tears fall into the paper and spread moisture from my nose to my mouth.

The door creaks open again. "Matt?"

"Yes?"

"You can come inside." A nurse holds the door open. Brittany turns and looks at me. She says nothing aloud but her face has a look of *What the hell is going on* across it.

"Sit, sit," says the nurse. So I do. I cautiously sit next to Brittany. "You won't hurt her or break anything," says the nurse, "and she's doing fine."

Brittany smiles through her fear. "Hi." A tear runs down her cheek. "They said the baby is okay."

"Hi. And so are you." Leaning forward, I kiss her forehead. *I sure hope so.*

4:15

Brittany squeezes my hand until my fingertips bleach white.

"Do you feel anything?" asks the doctor.

"No," she says. She squeezes harder.

"No," I say.

"All right," he says to the crew of 15 or so, "I'm going to make the cut. Hopefully we deliver this little girl quickly. Then I'll get her closed up. Everyone ready?"

The teams answer in clockwise order.

NICU team – ready!

Delivery nurse – ready!

Anesthesiologists – ready!

Nurses – ready!

"Here we go." He looks over the sheet at Brittany and me. "You'll see your baby in a just a minute. Let me know if you feel anything." He dips back behind the curtain. "Cutting. There she is. Move this to the side. Can you grab that? Have her. Closing her up."

The nurse walks around the sheet, leans forward, and shows us our three-pound alien.

"She's beautiful," I say. Tears stream down my

face and soak my mask.

Brittany sobs as our baby Liliana's head touches her own, forehead-to-forehead. "Look at all that hair!" she says.

She's got a head of hair like Magnum PI.

But her hairline runs down past her neck, over her shoulders, and down her back.

We created a tiny werewolf.

She's gorgeous.

The NICU team surrounds Liliana and work her like a pit crew at Daytona. "Vitals look good," says one of the nurses. "We're taking her up."

The doctor taps my shoulder. "You can come with us or you can stay here."

I look down at my wife, still spread across the operating table, crying. The smell of burning skin fills the room. She smiles at me. "Make sure she's okay. Go with her. I'll be okay."

The NICU team unlocks the incubator's wheels. They dart out of the OR's double doors, all running next to it. I follow.

As the doors close, the delivery doctor calls out, "Time of cut?"

"Four-fifteen."

"Time of delivery?"

"Four-fifteen."

"Time of closure?"

"Four-fifteen."

"Not bad," says the doc as the door seals shut.

WELCOME TO THE N.I.C.U.

The NICU team rolls Lil's incubator through another set of double doors as I sign in at the front desk. A woman hands me a thin hospital bracelet. "Don't lose this," she says, "you'll wear this until your baby is discharged."

"How long will that be?"

"Long as it takes. The doctors and nurses will walk you through it all. I'll walk you in now." She stands from behind her desk and guides me by the arm through the same doors. Noise blares out as the doors unseal. Beeps, bells, and chimes cry out like in some futuristic clock shop. We walk in.

"Your baby – "

"Liliana."

"Your baby Liliana is already in her new spot. We try to keep them in one spot while they're here. Like a little home for her."

Incubators line the walls like parked cars, each with about ten feet between them. Parents stand at some of them, changing diapers talking baby gibberish. They glance up at me as Liliana's team shouts out her stats and clears her lungs. The commotion is as chaotic as a bazaar. Yet, many of the babies sleep, unaware of the swirl around them.

The beeps, chimes, and dings blast out from the various monitors that surround each baby. They're set up like the spaceship in *Alien* – crude in build, sophisticated in technology. And many of the babies look more alien than human, like they'd burst through mom's chest and lay down in their new pods.

After a while the chaos around my Lil settles down and a nurse approaches me. "She's doing fine. She's three pounds and six ounces. We have a few more tests to run – all normal – so you are more than welcome to go back to see your wife. Come back in about 45 minutes and we'll give you a proper welcome."

I walk up to Lil's incubator and place my hand next to her. My hand is the same length as her body. Her little chest flutters up and down and her lips pucker. She's sprawled out like she's tanning. I put my fingertip into her hand and she closes her fingers around it. "I'll be right back. I have to check on Mommy," I say, and smile at her.

"She's in great hands. Best in the state. We'll see you in a few."

I blow Lil a kiss and leave the NICU.

AFTERBIRTH

Brittany sits propped in her hospital bed in the recovery area. She's smiling and no longer in a daze.

"She's three pounds, six ounces," I say. I kiss her lips. "She's beautiful. She's hairy. Very hairy."

Sitting on Brittany's bed, I notice a large cylindric container on the counter across from me. A reddish-brown goop fills the container and a giant piece of liver marinates inside the goop. At least it looks like liver. "What is that?" I ask.

"The placenta," says my mother-in-law, who sits on an empty OR bed across from us. "Nurse said they have to run tests on it."

"It's supposed to be good for your health," I say. I walk to the counter and pick up the container. "Looks delicious. A lot of people cook it and eat it." I stir the container. The afterbirth sloshes around. The placenta suctions to the sides and falls off. "I wouldn't cook it."

Brittany laughs. "There's something wrong with you."

"Definitely wouldn't cook it. I'd throw it into a protein shake. Nice and raw. Toss it in a blender with banana and milk. Maybe don't need the milk. Not with this womb juice. I bet if I eat your placenta, it'll be like *Highlander* and I absorb your intelligence. Finally, I'll be good at math."

"Stop," says Brittany, "you're making my stitches hurt," she laughs.

I walk back to her bed and kiss her. "Glad you're feeling more you. We can go see Lil in another twenty minutes."

"You'll be back in your room before that," says the nurse walking into our conversation. "And if you'd like, after the tests finish, I can ask the cafeteria throw this in a shake for you," she says. She jiggles the container.

"Thanks," I say. "Make a cup for each of us."

She winks at me over her shoulder. "We'll get you back into your room in a few minutes," she says, "and then you can head up to the NICU to see Liliana."

Autumn stands in front of us. "We met while you were on bed rest. And we introduced you to everything in here, but you probably forgot that already. So, we'll go through it again. I'm Autumn and I'm Liliana's lead nurse while she's on this level. There are three levels here. This is level three. As Liliana's strength improves, she'll move down to level two, then level one, then you'll take her home."

Autumn turns to face Lil in her incubator. "Liliana is going to be fine. We'll keep you updated on everything we do, need to do, or might have to do. If there's an urgent situation and you're not here, we'll call you. We'll move ahead if you don't answer. So, we'll need you to sign some forms to give us the permission to act quickly in her best interest."

Brittany, in a wheelchair still, squeezes my hand. "What kind of things would you have to do?"

"You never know. Every baby is different. In my twenty-plus years here, blood transfusions are the most common procedure. If we have to make that quick decision, we want to know we're doing right by her and you.

"Now onto you. You're going to want to be here twenty-four hours a day. You're going to feel guilty leaving. We take care of her, but we want to make sure you're healthy, too. Because you can't come in here if you're sick. We'll stop you at the door if you're so much as sniffling. Lil is three pounds. She doesn't need dad giving her a cold.

"Call if you're home and you want to check in. Call at any time. We'll talk to you as long as we're not busy with her or with one of the other babies. Leave a message if we don't answer and we'll call you back. It's important that you take care of yourselves. We'll help you get used to this. I know it's not easy."

At this point, I'd never thought about leaving the hospital without her. Never thought about walking around the house with Lil's bassinet empty, her room quiet. Brittany stares past Autumn, as if zoning out. She must be thinking about, too, dreading about the traumatic experience only a few days away.

Thin metal poles rise up above red and green glowing boxes. Cords run off the boxes and into the incubator and then into and onto Liliana. I follow each turning cord with my eyes and glare at the flashing numbers and blinking dots.

"Don't worry about all the gadgets behind me and

all the cords attached to Liliana," says Autumn. She catches me examining the crude-looking tech. "You'll get used to them and you'll know as much about them as I do before you leave."

Autumn steps behind Brittany's wheelchair and pushes her up to the incubator. Lil's swaddle blanket wraps from her chest to her feet. Her skinny arms, broken free, tuck under her chin. Brittany smiles a smile so strong it could warm the incubator itself.

"It will be a little while before you can hold her. But you can touch her. We recommend you keep it light for the next couple of days. We have what we call touch time. Every three hours we do all the things we need that require us to touch, move, or disturb Liliana. We'll change her diaper, change her cords, swap out equipment, feed her ... all that good stuff. Otherwise, we let her rest. If she moves around between two touch times, we let her go. Remember that she should still be inside, so this is all very fresh for her."

I want to hold her. Comfort her. Tell her that I'm here to protect her from now until my last breath. But she's so damn teeny and frail. The thought of touching her scares the crap out of me. What if I break her? I have a penchant for hulking things. I tear open cereal boxes and destroy reusable bags. I don't need to be handling my three-pound baby.

"I can't wait until you can hold her," I say to Brittany. She won't accidentally smash her.

THAT'S A DIAPER

Everything is miniature. The feeding tube's small enough to fit through an earring hole. The blood pressure collar too small to wrap around two of my fingers. And the diaper – the diaper is smaller than a pack of gum.

"Pick it up and open it out," says Autumn.

I stare at the teeny poop catcher. "That's really a diaper?"

"It is."

Open new diaper. Spread new diaper. Lie baby on new diaper. Unwrap old diaper. The old diaper is only wet. I roll it up, stick it together in a ball, and put it aside. Then I surround Lil's hips with the new diaper and tape it closed. Admiring my work, I lift her butt off the incubator floor. The diaper slides down her thin legs and hangs at her ankles.

"These are the smallest diapers they make. They're usually still too big for the kids in here. You have to roll the top and then tape," says Autumn.

"Way too big," I say and start over.

SIBLING VISITS

Diana has trekked to the hospital from an hour and a half away. The closest to us geographically, she visited when Brittany was bedridden in the hospital and now, she's checking in after Lil's birth. She's my older sister and even though we're no longer little kids, I still look up to her, both for advice and for comfort. We hug when she arrives at the front counter and I help check her in. Our embrace is grippy, I feel my fingertips curl around her shoulders. She's strong.

"Thank you so much," I say. We walk the long hallway from the hospital entrance to the maternity ward. She'll see Brittany first. She kisses Brittany and then we head to the NICU.

"Now, before we go in, we have to follow a strict routine," I say. I show her the sink and the soap and point to the soap that I use, the grittier one. "Feels like it's scraping the germs off," I say. "No one can go in there," I point to the NICU doors, "unless they're scrubbed in and covered." I hand her a gown and mask.

Dressed like we're performing an operation, we walk through the double-doors together and I feel my chest heave as I get excited to introduce her to my first daughter and her first niece. *This is not how I imagined it would be.* We loop around a nurse's station and I wave her toward Lil's incubator. *Then again, I didn't have any expectations. And now I'm already used to seeing Lil Bear this way.*

My eyes swell. "Lil, your Aunt Diana is here to meet you." I press my hand on Lil's incubator glass. "Diana, this is Lil." I can't help but hug my older sister again. No matter how much taller or heavier I am or how much older we both are, our hug is always the same, our arms wrapped around each other and my face burrowed in her shoulder. She's always looking out for her little brother.

Diana stays at the hospital a while and chats with Brittany and then leaves a couple hours later.

My younger sister, Maria, visits a few days later. She will forever be my little sister. She arrives and we go through a similar routine. I check her in, she sees Brittany, and then we dress for the NICU.

"Lil, your Aunt Maria is here to see you." I cry and see that Maria is doing the same. They're happy tears. And we hug in our own way. Maria leans sideways into my right shoulder and I wrap my right arm around her and she presses her head onto my shoulder and neck and we stand there quietly looking at Lil for a while. It's her way of saying *I'm here, brother.* It's my way of saying *everything is okay, sister, no need to worry.*

A few days later my younger brother visits the hospital. Same routine. Check-in and gear up for the NICU. He will forever be my baby brother, even though he towers over me and has outdone me in every way in life.

We walk into the NICU and look into Lil's incubator. "Lil, this is your Uncle Raymond." I cry harder than I had with my sisters. Raymond and I stand side-by-side and as I sob, he puts his arm around my shoulder and pulls me in closer and I sob some more.

UNFILTERED NURSE

Brittany and I sit on rolling chairs next to Lil's incubator. It's a busy morning. Alarms ring and nurses scurry back and forth. But nothing major. Lil is amazingly well. She sleeps and we stare at her, a daily occurrence.

We chatter with the nurses – another daily occurrence. They're here all the time and so are we, and damned if I don't get to know people. As the alarms quiet down, the nurses sit and stand around us. We're the only parents in the NICU.

"So, I have to ask … why do you come here so late at night?" Mel, one of the nurses, looks at me. She sits in her own roller chair and fills out papers as she leans on a clipboard.

"I travel. I fly to Minneapolis on Monday morning and fly home Thursday afternoon."

"A lot?"

Like all the other nurses, Mel is an angel. But unlike the other nurses, she tends to speak her mind. We laugh at her because her mind is normally harmless.

"Yup. Every week."

"So, you've been traveling ever since Brittany's been here?"

"I stopped for a week and then went back to traveling," I say.

Her eyes pierce me with a puzzled yet concerned look. Like, *how dare you leave these two vulnerable ladies here while you're off globetrotting.* "And so you show up here on Thursday nights," she says.

Guerly sees the foot-in-mouth unfolding. She must be used to this just as she's used to hearing the preemie's alarms ring. "Mel, he needs to work." Guerly moves closer to us as Mel moves her chair closer to me. Guerly is attempting an intercept.

"So," says Mel, "how long will you travel now that you have a little daughter?"

"I'm traveling now so that I can save my paternity time," I say. I look at Brittany. Her head is tilted and she's looking at Lil, pretending like none of this is happening and letting me get grilled. Her grin stretches out of her mask. *What a jerk.*

"How long will you have paternity for?" asks Mel.

"I'll take one week as soon as Lil comes home and then I'll take another week later on. I might take a vacation week early, too, just so I'm home."

Mel can't believe it. "You mean to tell me that

after all this, you'll take one or two weeks and then just head off again and leave your daughter behind?"

Behind Mel, Guerly's eyes bulge in disbelief. "Mel, he's gotta work," says Guerly.

"I know, but he's so far away. He could work anywhere. He could work in New York."

"It can take just as long to get in and out of the city," I say. "And it's more stressful. And I don't get any travel points." Now I'm enjoying messing with Mel. "Brittany and Lil will be fine. If they need something I can be home in four hours. They'll make do."

"But are you going to stay with this job?" asks Mel. "Or are you looking for something closer?"

"I enjoy my work," I say.

"He does," says Brittany. "Being away has brought us closer."

Mel is completely puzzled.

"And what's nice is that I don't have to be in Minneapolis. I go there because Target is a client. I could have other clients and fly to other cities. I could fly to San Francisco every week. That would be pretty cool," I say.

"But that's a six-hour flight," says Mel. "I can't believe you'd do that."

“Think of all the points,” I say. “Brittany and Lil will be fine. They’ll manage.”

“You’re going to miss your daughter’s entire life so that you can collect travel points?” she says. “Just for a few credits?”

Guerly swoops in, grabs the back of Mel’s chair and pulls her away from us and to the other side of the room. “Mel, you can’t say that,” she says to her.

“I … I don’t get it.”

“We can tell,” says Guerly. “Stay here for a while.” Guerly walks back to us laughing. “I’m sorry. She’s an idiot.”

“That’s okay,” I say, laughing. “It was hysterical. And I can’t blame her. I’ve asked myself the same questions a million times.”

An alarm rings and the nurses break away from us. Brittany and I hold hands and peer into Lil’s incubator. She sleeps soundly. And I wonder, how will I be there for her when I travel so much? I peak at Brittany. How will I be there for her or Lil … when I won’t actually be there?

GOING HOME ALONE

We're going home. I jam the last of the stuffed animals into our Civic's trunk. I load in the flowers, balloons, and bags of clothes. There's no car seat. *Don't say anything stupid.*

A few minutes earlier, the NICU nurse assured us the first time going home was hardest. "After that, it doesn't hurt so much. Honest truth," she said. "Call during the next changing time," she glanced at her watch, "about 1am." We looked down at our Liliana, wrapped in a blanket, wires and hoses snaking around her and into her nose and throat and bellybutton. She was beautiful, a bit hairy, and just under three pounds. Our Lil Bear.

Brittany waits in a wheelchair under the hospital's overhang. I pull the car around and help her slide onto the passenger seat. She winces and presses a hand to her new abdominal wound. "New parents aren't supposed to leave without their baby. This is unnatural," she says.

I say nothing. I say nothing stupid.

It's gray and a drizzle blankets the windshield, just enough to need the wipers, but not enough to keep them on. I manually flick them on and off as we drive south on Route 18.

On. Don't say something stupid.

Off. Don't say something stupid.

On. God, please keep me from being an idiot.

Finally, we pull into our driveway, our headlights shining through our small house's bay window and into the dark house. Our dogs' faces pop up and peek out at us and then disappear. I hop out of the car and guide Brittany through the front door. Our dogs Sandi and Patty greet us with their wet noses. Brittany fishes through her bag and pulls out a small white blanket with blue and red stripes. "They need to smell the baby," she says and lets them sniff.

We settle in. It's eleven and we want to stay awake until we can call and check on Lil.

"Can we watch something funny?" asks Brittany. She props herself up on our sectional.

"Sure. I'm making coffee," I say and walk into the kitchen. "You know," I say, "it's pretty quiet in here without a …"

You've got to be shitting me. Stop! Put it all back in your mouth, you fucking idiot. Too late.

"… without a baby." I double over and wail uncontrollably. Brittany weeps.

I slither onto the couch. "I was trying so hard not to say anything dumb," I say still crying. "I said the dumbest thing possible."

Brittany laughs through her tears. "What the hell is wrong with you?" she says. We burst out laughing.

I make coffee twice more that night. Both times, I cry my eyes out then laugh my ass off.

HOLDING YOU (KANGAROO)

"You're here late," says Autumn as I walk through the NICU's mechanical double doors. She sits at the desk outside of the entryway to the tiny people.

"Delayed flight. By a lot."

"It's almost touch time. And good news. You can kangaroo her."

"Brittany told me this afternoon. She was ecstatic on the phone. That's why I came straight from the airport even though it's almost 3am. Didn't want to wait until tomorrow morning."

Autumn stands up. "I'll come in with you, but then I'll leave you alone."

We scrub our hands at the sink, my skin cracked from the constant washing. The burn is worth it if it lets me see Lil and keeps her healthy. I slip on my yellow gown and mask and we walk through the doors and head right to Lil's incubator.

"Come sit," says Autumn.

So I do.

"She'll still have her lines and tubes, so you can't walk around. But you can rock. You can move her position if it gets uncomfortable." She pulls Lil – still about three pounds – from her glass house and slides her onto my forearms. She unbuttons my top two dress shirt buttons for me. "Now, gently slide her down your shirt. Her blanket can unwind a bit. You want her skin on your skin."

She's swaddled like a taco. I awkwardly lift her up, still unsure of my ability to handle something so fragile and guide her down my shirt. "She's so warm."

"She's incubated. Now I'll leave you two alone. I'll be doing rounds if you need anything."

I sit in the rocking chair next to Lil's incubator and Lil snuggles against my chest. We're surrounded by other babies and alarms ring out, but for a moment it feels like we're by ourselves, cocooned in our own world.

"You have to gain weight," I tell her. "Mom can't wait to take you home. Neither can I. But I'm also terrified I'll break you."

Her eyes close and she smooshes her face into my chest hair.

"Sorry about that. Not as nice as Mom's chest."

Lil is as hot as a towel that's just come out of the dryer. It feels comfortable after a few minutes.

I finally feel like a dad.

"So, this is what it's all about," I say, "there's

nothing better." We rock in the chair and I sing *What a Wonderful World* until my eyes close. Not sleeping. Enjoying.

SETTLE DOWN, SETTLE DOWN

Late nights become regular, especially on Thursdays. I intentionally book the 8pm flight from Minneapolis to Newark and roll into the NICU at around 1:30am. It's quiet. Lil and I sit and talk and sing. She doesn't react much to my updates about work. Songs move her. She buries her head into my chest as I sing *You are My Sunshine, Alberta,* and *San Francisco Bay Blues.* She's either saying she loves me or covering her ears to avoid my voice. The latter is probable.

We rock. Relaxed on the chair, my left hand cups her tiny butt and my right holds her back. The NICU is calm. Regardless of the fear, these nights are a respite.

Beep. Beep. Beep. Ding. Lil's alarm bells scream out. She squirms in my arms. Her heartbeat accelerates faster and faster. A nurse jogs over and turns off the chimes. Lights still flash red and yellow. "We'll keep an eye on her. This happens." She walks away.

What do I do? First real parenting moment and I'm frozen. I pull her in tighter. "Settle down," I say. "Settle down and follow my breath." I breathe deep and lift her entire body with my chest. "Breathe with me. Settle down. Settle down." Her breathing slows to match mine. Her heart rate drops from 110 to 65. The red-light switches to green. Our slow breathing steadies. Lil opens her eyes and looks at me. She closes them again and falls to sleep. I close my eyes. I'll leave at three, as I doze off.

THE SONGS WE SING

On those quiet nights, Lil and I sit together on a chair and listen to our favorite tunes. They're really my favorite tunes. But I promised myself that as a dad I would introduce her to the best music, to the music that I grew up loving and listening to – none of that crap I hear on the radio today.

We rock in the chair, Lil tucked into my shirt like we're a couple of koalas. "Okay, what should we put on?" I thumb through my playlists and albums on my phone. "A little late for Zeppelin. Maybe later. How about something softer?" I scroll around and land on Louis Armstrong. "This is good, Lil," I say and tap *What a Wonderful World.*

We swing forward and backward to the beat and I tap my foot. "He plays the trumpet. He was good. So was Dizzy. And Dizzy had these big puffy cheeks. I played the trombone for a long time. Not as many famous trombone players."

The song ends and I sing her the final words, "yes, I think to myself, what a wonderful world." The music stops and I look down at her and rub her cheek with my index finger. "It's true you know," I whisper, "Sure you're in here. But you'll get out of here and just getting to hold you and sit with you late at night, well, there's nothing more wonderful."

I scroll through my list again. "How about some famous guitarists?" I ask. "Clapton?" I flick on his unplugged album and play *Running on Faith* and I hum the slide guitar opening for her. She doesn't move. She just lies against my chest and breathes. But her alarms are quiet and so I assume it must be working – she must enjoy this time with me. I certainly enjoy this time with her.

FIRST BOTTLE

The challenge seems simple – drink 15 ounces of milk in a sitting. That's less than a shot at the bar. But it's not so simple for Lil. The bottle dwarfs her like everything else and sprawls from her mouth to her belly button.

"We thawed out about fifteen ounces of Mom's milk," says the nurse, "but we don't expect her to drink it all. We'd love her to but want to be realistic. We also don't want to waste Mom's precious milk."

Brittany smiles. She's making milk but not as easily as she hoped. The breast pump sounds like a meat grinder. I wonder what it's like, but I don't want to try it and lose a nipple.

"Mom will feed her first," says the nurse.

Brittany smiles again. She's been waiting for this. Lil was born three weeks ago. A week passed before we could hold her. Now three weeks in and she's only been tube fed. These are the milestones we'll never forget that other parents may never remember. Bottle feeding for them is just how it goes. It's a victory for us and it's a signal that we may go home as a family soon. Brittany sits in the chair next to Lil's incubator and flattens her scrubs, patting the material down.

The nurse pulls Lil from her incubator, guiding the handful of cords and tubes so as not to get caught or tangled. She lays her in Brittany's lap. "Here's the milk, dear," says the nurse, handing Brittany the bottle. Brittany scooches her butt back a bit and slides her elbow onto the chair's arm. Lil lies comfortably in Brittany's nook.

Brittany lightly presses the nipple across Lil's lips. At first Lil scrunches her face, unaware of what deliciousness she's turning down. Brittany presses again. Lil takes the bottle.

"It may take her some time," says the nurse. "Babies this age are still in the womb and don't need this skill yet."

"She's drinking!" says Brittany. Brittany's face stretches happy. Her eyes shimmer and her nose crinkles. Only twice in the past three weeks has she looked fully happy. First holding Lil and now feeding her. She's a "normal" mom – what she imagined when we decided to have kids and what she'd read about in all those bullshit *What to Expect* books.

I want to feed Lil. Instead, I sit next to Brittany and watch her moment.

ONE MONTH

One-month birthdays are joyous celebrations. You see the pictures online – the still alien-looking baby leaning against a teddy bear. Parents high-five their survival skills. They've not slept in 30-days, but they haven't broken the kid.

Everything is different for us. We're grateful that Lil moved out of the incubator. But tubes and cords flow out of her like she's an explosive. This doesn't stop Brittany. She will celebrate this one-month milestone. And why not? She deserves it.

Brittany lays outfits across the bottom of the crib and holds them against Lil. Lil fusses and pulls at her feeding tube. Brittany's kept it together and made the best of being at the NICU every day for a month. It's tiring ... but a blessing. We've had more time to prep the house. The baby's room is still empty every night. Soon that will change.

Brittany smooshes a pink number one sticker onto Lil's white outfit. She pulls a headband with a giant blue bow over her head. The bow is the same size as her face and could double as a visor. She looks adorable. Brittany's done a fine job.

The feeding tube sticks out from Lil's nostril. She pulls at it. "I would love to get rid of it, too," says Brittany, "at least for pictures." With that Lil yanks the tube out of her nose. The nurse, standing close by, picks up the tube. "I'll get this right back in," she says and does so in seconds. Lil pulls it out again. "Well, I guess you don't want that anymore," says the nurse.

Brittany frowns through her smile. "Can we leave it out for her pictures?"

"You know what … she's taking the bottle right?"

"She is."

"She's done with it," says the nurse.

"For good?" I ask.

"She takes the bottle. You don't want this up her nose anymore. She doesn't want this up her nose anymore. Why have it up her nose? We'll keep it out for the day and see how she does." The nurse removes the tube from Lil's crib and lays it in a nearby sink. "I'll take your picture, too. What a beautiful family." Brittany hands her the big camera.

The nurse clicks away. We stand, Brittany beaming with excitement. Lil coos. She small grins and pokes out her tongue. She's hit a milestone. She knows it somehow. She's proud of herself. She told us to get that damn hose out of her tiny nose.

One month into family-hood. The past four weeks have been tough. Today though, I smile for the camera. I smile for Brittany and her getting closer to normalcy. I smile for Lil and her clear nostril. I smile because regardless of how difficult this is, I wouldn't change it. I don't think.

PASSING TESTS

Brittany and I stand in front of Lil's crib. She's graduated from an incubator to a crib. She's a real infant now. Almost.

"Before you're allowed to go home," says Autumn, "all three of you have to pass an array of tests."

"Tests?"

"You think we'll just let you prance out of here?"

"No," I say.

"Mom and Dad, you'll have to take CPR and baby Heimlich. There are a few other things we check off that you've already passed. Dad, you haven't dropped Lil yet and you know how to change a diaper."

"Not well," I say.

Autumn keeps talking. "Lil will be monitored by another group overnight, make sure she's always breathing. She'll also have to be monitored while she's buckled in a car seat. Can't take her home if she can't breathe in a car seat. Make sense?"

"Yup," we say.

We sit at a table alongside another couple who's hoping to bring home their preemie, too. A coach stands over us and plops two dolls on the tabletop. "These are your kids," she says. "By the end of the hour, you'll be able to save your actual baby's life, should you need to. We'll go over how to clear your baby's throat, how to smack food out of their throat, and how to do CPR."

I hold the doll in my hands and tuck it into my chest like a football. "Do all new parents get this training?" I ask.

"Nope," says the coach. "Only NICU parents."

"So, parents with regular babies are just supposed to know this stuff?"

"Yup."

For the first time, I'm happy we are in the NICU.

"Your baby is choking," says the coach, "pick her up, turn her on her stomach on the palm of your hand. With your other palm, smack her between her shoulder blades." I hold the doll and tap her back like she's a bag of chips that I'm afraid to crush. "Give her a good whack," says the coach. "Don't be afraid." My wife watches as I thwack the doll right on target. The doll's head smacks the table and she falls out of my hand.

"Crap, I'm going to fail," I say picking up the baby. I pass the doll to Brittany.

“That’s okay,” says Brittany, “you’ll never be alone with them anyway.”

“I’ll pretend like I didn’t see that,” says the coach. “Try not to concuss her this time.”

“We’ll be here longer than an hour,” I say.

GOING HOME TOGETHER

We strap Lil into her car seat. She's wrapped in a warm onesie and a teeny beanie, keeping her temperature up. She looks like a doll. The seat swallows her making her barely visible.

"Ready to go?" asks Ercillia. She's been Lil's main nurse on the lower level. She's beaming. Another baby is graduating out of the NICU. The earth angels have saved another life.

"We are," says Brittany from a wheelchair. "But we will miss you." She's right. We've spent the past five weeks at the hospital with Lil. But by talking to the doctors, nurses, and volunteers every day, we came to know many of them like family.

Ercillia unbuckles Lil from her car seat, pulls her out, and lays her on Brittany's lap. "The wheelchair is protocol," she says, "and you deserve to hold her as you leave." She slides behind the wheelchair and pushes Brittany toward the NICU door. "Say goodbye." The other nurses stand at the door. We hug and cry as we cross over the threshold into the hallway. "Remember, we're still here. Call if you have any questions."

Autumn walks toward us from down the hall and opens her arms wide as she gets closer.

"Congratulations," she says. "Lil was strong from the beginning. You have everything you need?" We hug.

"Think so," says Brittany. "I've been waiting for this."

"We know," says Autumn.

Ercillia walks us down the hall away from the NICU and toward the front door. We've done it. We left the hospital empty-handed every night. At home, we lived with an empty child's room and crib. We called the NICU every morning at 2am to find out if Lil peed, pooped, or cried. We endured an emotional torture. Now that's over.

We'll be a regular family. As regular as possible. Even though we won't.

Most parents don't have monitors hooked up to their babies at home. We will.

Most parents don't have to keep their babies away from other people's germs. We will.

Most parents don't have to track their baby's bodily functions. We will.

But we'll do it at home – together.

NOT A DOLL

Brittany and I are afraid to take Lil anywhere. Not because we doubt ourselves as parents, but because we're afraid how others will react. We've seen the old-person-versus-baby behavior with our nephew and niece: old person sees baby, old person touches baby, old person gives germs to baby. For whatever reason old people can't help but put their filthy hands on newborns. Doesn't matter where they are or what the occasion. A mom could be pushing a stroller past an old man in a supermarket and the old man will think it perfectly fine to step in front of the stroller and jam his old fingers into the newborn's hand. And the face. Old folks love newborn faces.

But we can't stay inside forever. After a couple of weeks at home, we decide we need to get out and at least have some dinner. We dress ourselves and Brittany dresses Lil and hooks up her monitor and makes sure her cords are nice and secure, so they don't alarm while we're eating. Then we head to Graziano's – our favorite local Italian restaurant.

We've been eating here for a few years and Brittany's parents have been dining here for decades.

We know the owners and the staff and it's a bit like having dinner at your aunt's house. Of course, everyone we know who's working will want to see Lil and that's fine. We happily show off our tiny treasure. For a moment, we feel like real parents, even though I'm holding the monitor box. Instead of hiding it, I explain how it works to the waitresses.

And then it happens.

We're eating our dinner and Lil's car seat is propped up on a flipped-over highchair. An older couple, having finished their dinner at a nearby table, walks by our table and the woman glances down at Lil. "Oh my. Look, look," she says to her husband.

They stop and hover and barely even look at us. "She's small," says the husband.

Don't touch her. Don't put your smelly, old hands on her.

I peak at Brittany. She's looking at the old couple, smiling, but I can see through her smile. She's thinking the same thing as me.

Don't put your mothball fingers near my Lil.

I don't know if I'm smiling or baring my teeth.

"She's just so precious. She's so tiny," says the old woman. "We saw you hold her and for a second there we thought she was a doll. She's just so small she doesn't look real." The old hag puts her index finger down onto the car seat near Lil's swaddled feet.

Don't touch Lil's fucking car seat with your old skin.

"She is real," says Brittany. Somehow, she's still smiling. "She's about five pounds. This is the first time we have her out because we have to be careful exposing her to too many germs. She's a preemie."

Get the fuck away from my kid, Mother Hubbard.

"How is everything, guys?" Our waitress Donna asks and pushes in front of the old couple. "Excuse me," she says.

"Good luck with her. Congratulations," says the old woman. They leave the restaurant.

"Thanks" says Brittany to Donna.

"I could tell they were bothering you," Donna says. "You okay, hun?" she asks me.

"Oh yeah," I say, "I was fine the whole time."

Brittany looks at me. "Liar."

LIL SHIT

Preemie diapers are the size of a pack of gum. The entire diaper seems like it can hold a sneeze worth's of pee or poop. But so far so good. I fold the diaper's edges over and press the sticky tabs down and get Lil ready for a big family outing. "We're going to Target," I tell her. "You're not going inside. Place is littered with old people." I dress her and settle her in the car seat. Brittany, Lil, and I drive to Brick, New Jersey to our closest Target.

It's busy and so I park a few rows away from the entrance. "Okay," says Brittany, "I only have a few things to get, so I should be fast. Think you've got it?"

I give her a *you think I can't handle watching my daughter in a car seat* look. "Baber," I say, "come on."

"Okay. Well, call if you need me." She walks away from the car and disappears into the cavernous store.

I look into the backseat and peak at Lil. "How you doing back there? Good? How about some music?"

I turn on Clapton's *Unplugged* album and skip to the song *Alberta* and slap the steering wheel and sing to her. There's a mirror that faces her so I can look in the rearview and see her, check that she's okay. She smiles and then squirms in her seat and smooshes her cheeks together. "You dancing back there?"

We sing a few more songs.

A foul odor wafts to the front seat and punches itself up my nose. "What the hell is that? Damn, Lil." I roll down the window and let the fresh air fight the stink. But it's unbearable. Turning around to face Lil, I look in the backseat. "Kiddo, what the hell – "

Lil smiles. She plays with a rattle ball and laughs as it jingles. But her hand is covered in a brown-green slime. "What's that? Did you put your hand in your diaper?"

Lil squeals as if enjoying her cheekiness. Her hands disappear into her car seat and when she pulls them out, they're both covered in brown-green slime. "What are you doing? How did you – "

I get out of the car and walk around to her side and open her door. "What is going on, kiddo. Your outfit looks clean. And you shouldn't be able to get your hands into your diaper." I lean her over a bit. Holy shit.

Shit. She's covered in shit. The notorious baby blowout. Lil's done it. In her car seat. In the Target parking lot. "Okay, I've got this. First, I have to wipe those hands." So, I take out the baby wipes and clean off her hands. "Now don't touch anything."

I unbuckle her and lean her to the side. Shit. Shit is pooling in the bottom of the car seat. Shit's splattered up her back, down her legs, and onto the back of her neck. She's lying in a puddle of shit. Shit, what am I going to do?

I lift her up and hold her away from me. "Maybe I unbutton your outfit and pull it up over your head. No, then your face will be covered in shit. What if I unbutton it and pull it down? No, then everything else will be covered in shit." Panic sets in.

I look at her and I stare at the shit. Lil just smiles. "You're really making me look bad here, kiddo. What am I going to do?" My chest tightens and sweat drips down my forehead and my hands clam up. I hold her out in front of me. "I don't know what to do."

I spin my head around and scan the parking lot, hoping miraculously someone with blowout experience comes along.

No one.

I glance around again and see Brittany walking toward me carrying a few bags. "Baber! Help!" I couldn't watch Lil for the 15 minutes Brittany ran into the store. Fail. But screw it. "Help!"

She walks up to us and shakes her head. "What happened?"

"Lil shit everywhere," I say. "It's on everything. She was even playing with it."

"God, that stinks. Lil, did you give Dad a hard time?"

Lil smirks like she understands.

Brittany examines the situation and I watch her process it all. I can see her mind work. Her head tilts a bit to the left and then to the right and her eyes slim and then her lips press together and smile. She knows exactly what she's going to do. She walks to the back of the car and pulls out plastic shopping bags and plucks the baby wipes out of her handbag. "All right. Let's get you clean."

And then she meticulously executes her plan, wiping Lil, changing her clothes, and cleaning the car seat… seamlessly. I watch in awe at her motherhood. *How the hell does she know how to do this?*

30 minutes later, we're driving home. Lil's in the backseat sleeping, tired from her shitstorm. "That was impressive," I say.

"Thanks. You did a great job," says Brittany.

"Shut up," I say.

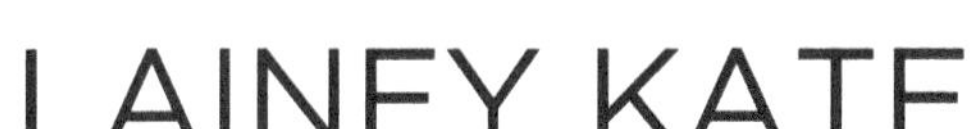
LAINEY KATE

A PISTOL FROM THE START

Brittany's pregnancy with Lainey 3 years later is high-risk from the beginning. Go into labor 10-weeks early one time and doctors treat you differently. So Brittany spends more time at the OB than she does with me. And she has to get 3D ultrasounds a few times a month, so the doctors can spot any abnormalities with the baby or with Brittany early. And so that we can see how much the thing growing inside my wife looks like a mushy version of the alien from *Space Balls*.

It's week 20. Brittany and I sit in the car outside the 3D ultrasound office.

"How many kids do you want?" she asks.

It's a question I hadn't really considered.

"I would love four girls, each two to three years apart," she says.

I smile because I envision being a dad to four girls and it seems perfect. "I can see that. No boys?"

"I like girls. Of course, a boy would be fine, but I like girls," says Brittany.

"Okay, but I'm going to do all the boy things with one of them and then she'll probably wind up being ugly and butch," I say.

A WHATTA?

We agree to having two more girls and walk into the doctor's office. A while later, Brittany lies on the exam table, her shirt lifted exposing her stomach. "Stop looking at me like that," she says.

"Sorry," says my wife to the ultrasound tech, "my husband is an idiot."

The tech measures the baby's body parts, her left hand guiding a wand over Brittany's lubed skin and her right hand tapping a keyboard. She does this for fifteen minutes. "I have to get the doctor," she says and leaves us in the room.

"Something's wrong," says Brittany. "She got up and left. That's never happened before."

"Everything is fine," I say. I have no idea what's happening, but I have no idea about most things.

The doctor and tech walk back in together. She sits in her chair and works the wand over Brittany's belly again. The doctor hunches over, staring at the screen. "There," says the tech.

"Yes, yes," says the doctor.

They turn to face us. "It's a good thing you come here," says the doctor. "A regular ultrasound may not have picked this up. First, the baby is fine. Perfectly fine."

I actually breathe a sigh of relief. But if the baby is fine, why the hell are you in here?

"Brittany, you have something called placenta accreta. Let me explain. Normally, the placenta hovers close to the uterine wall. With accreta, the placenta becomes attached to the uterine wall. There are various types. With the least dangerous, it only attaches to the wall. But it can also grow out and around the uterus or grow out of the uterus and attach to the other internal organs. Right now you have the least dangerous case... but we have to monitor it."

"What does that mean?" asks Brittany. The tech lowers her head.

"Well, first you have to come here more often. Second, this is now an extremely high-risk pregnancy. This is still one of the main reasons women die during childbirth. But the fact that we caught it puts us in the driver seat, to an extent. We will call your OB and they will get in touch with all the other doctors who need to work at your scheduled C-section. For your safety and to increase your chances of survival, we recommend a hysterectomy." He pauses. "It's your choice if you want to attempt to keep your uterus.

But there aren't many doctors in the country who've delivered women with accreta. Trying to save the uterus adds risk on top of risk."

Looks like we're stopping at two girls. Brittany's hands cover her eyes as she heaves crying, lying helpless on the table. And there's nothing I can do. We just talked about four girls. She let me into her dream and her own body crushed it. And now we have to worry about her dying and not getting to see Lil grow up. I take her hand and squeeze.

"I'll leave you for a few minutes. Then we'll have to go over the plan," says the doctor. He walks out of the room while I hug Brittany in an attempt to console her, to let her know all will be okay. But I don't know many things.

PHONE CALLS TO FAMILY ... AGAIN

Here we are again. There's an obligation to call my family – my parents, sisters, and brother – to tell them that Brittany's pregnancy is now a crap shoot, that we need an army of specialists in the delivery room with us, that accreta is the top reason women die during childbirth, that Brittany could hemorrhage at any time, that the baby isn't guaranteed to make it, especially if Brittany hemorrhages too soon.

Sitting in our SUV and scrolling through my phone, I call my parents individually. They're working. Then I call my sisters. Then my brother. Once again – like when Brittany went into the hospital early with Lil – my eyes fill with tears each call. But this time it's slightly different. I don't want to lose my wife. The old debate about whether you should want someone in your life or need someone in your life is horseshit. When you're dating you might want your girlfriend in your life. When you're married and love each other, you need one another. Rip that apart and you're not fine, not able to jump back into life with a perky stride.

I cry a lot while telling my dad. "Brittany will be fine," he says. "The baby will be fine." He says it over and over again. At first, it's a bit annoying – shit, she's going to bleed out next week and I'm going to lose her and the baby and be a single father. He says it a few more times, "They'll both be okay."

It's hard to tell if it's his way of coping with the news or if it's his way of calming me down. Doesn't matter, the latter starts to work. "They'll be fine," he says again in a steady voice.

Wiping the tears from my cheeks with my forearm, I half smile. "You're right, Dad, they will be okay. The doctors are great and they caught it. That's half the battle." He's convinced me to convince myself that all is well. "Thanks, Dad, I have to call Raymond now."

We hang up and I call my brother. I walk to the deck in our yard to sit and let the fresh air hit my face and dry any remnants of being an emotional basket case. I'm calm. I'm accepting of reality. "Raymond, I have to tell you something … Brittany has something called accreta and – " I bawl. Dammit, I've not even sat down yet.

LOVING TWO

The excitement of having two girls morphs into fear of losing Brittany and the baby. That morphs into a laundry list of fears that I attempt to either forget about or answer with quick Google searches – a terrible idea. I can see the fear in my mind, a giant black cloud of doom enveloping all the happy thoughts.

It's 5am. I sit at our kitchen table with the light dimmed, my notebook and laptop out. *How will I love two kids?* I write in my notebook. This fear plagues me most, aside from the death of my wife, of course.

I pseudo-parent. Because I spend the majority of my time on the road, I don't have to parent like Brittany does. I'm not there for every waking issue. Lil knows this even though she's young. She sees me as the fun man who is around in short spurts and puts her to bed.

But she doesn't even know how many nights I put her to bed because she doesn't understand the concept of a week yet.

I write all of this in my notebook and drink my

black coffee and stare out into the living room and terrify myself.

With so little time home, how will I split it between two kids? How will I look at two kids and love them both equally?

Our black Lab Patty licks my hand and scares me and I look down at her and scratch her thick neck fur. "Oh crap. I love you, too." Our yellow Lab Sandi snores in the living room. "Oh no."

The kitchen lights brighten and Brittany turns the corner and yawns. "What are you doing?" she asks.

CHOICE

As a teenager, I attended the Pro-Life March in Washington, bused there by my Catholic high school. A little guy in a big town making my young voice heard. I even made the local news and answered some questions for a rookie reporter. "This is a wonderful event," I said, "because thousands of people from all over the country join together to stop abortion."

What a fool. What would you tell your younger self? is a question I hear a lot these days. Brittany and I sit in the kitchen at our table and read through a stack of papers. The delivery doctors asked us to fill these out and return them. The papers document our answer to a life altering question – who lives and who dies? Do we prefer to save the baby and let Brittany, my love, my wife, the mother of our three-year-old, die? Do we save Brittany and let our still growing kind-of-baby die? Does our decision change when Brittany's 28 weeks pregnant? How about at 29 weeks? Each week requires a choice and a signature.

We know we have to fill these out. We know, regardless of what we sign on the papers, that Brittany may die. At this point, I'd only thought about that and not considered the risk to the baby.

What would I tell my younger self? Nothing. I'd walk up to myself in Washington and punch myself in my face. How dare I take a stand on something that I had zero understanding of? How dare I believe that I had the wisdom to tell others how to choose life or death – but only life – because I was better, because I went to Catholic school? I'd walk up to myself, pull my shirt over my head, and punch myself in the dumb fucking face.

Brittany cries at the table. "How am I supposed to make these decisions?" I stand up beside her and wrap my arms around her shoulders. We cry, pushing the stack of hell to the side. "We'll do this another time," I say. When is a good time to decide if my wife gets to watch Liliana grow up? Never. Yet we have to fill out the papers.

GODDAMN PONYTAILS

The three of us sit on the couch. Lil gets ready for bed. Brittany smothers her in lotion and brushes and braids her curly hair. I watch as Brittany's hands work without thought. She's a mom. She innately knows how to carve Lil's thick locks, twirling them up and under and over, until there's a smooth braid.

They watch another episode of *Sarah and Duck*. I stare at Brittany's hands. How the hell am I going to do this? I've tried fixing up Lil's hair. She looked like one of those dread-locked dogs. I can't braid. I can barely brush. How am I going to do this for two girls? How am I going to raise two girls myself? I panic.

"You can't leave me," I whisper to Brittany.

"Huh?" Lil leans back into Brittany's lap. She's tired.

"I can't braid her hair. I will be terrible at this by myself."

This is the first time I've shared my concern with Brittany. I let her know I need her support.

She smiles and kisses Lil's damp head. "You're a great dad. And you'd be fine, even with braids. Though in my will I'll probably write that my mom has to do their hair every night."

We watch the rest of the show. Lil leans on Brittany and Brittany leans on me. A trio of love. I glance at the braid. We'll either stay a trio, become a quartet, or reduce to a duo. I enjoy what I have on the couch right now. I'll handle the damn ponytail later.

SHOWER CRY

Happiness, or the perception of it, is my number one goal every day. The fear and the worry sneak around. Suppressed. It's as if I press against a door with all my strength, but a beast pushes from the other side, hoping to destroy those I love. Humor is my weapon. Suppression is my armor. Brittany appreciates my ability to drop comical lines into regular conversation. But she does occasionally say, "You don't take anything seriously."

I can be serious. At the same time, screw it. We're here once. We can't redo much. Why not laugh while you're living, even if current events are shitty.

As Brittany and I left the high-risk doctor's office that day, I vowed to inject humor into everything. Brittany should never need to lift me up. Aside from the braid meltdown, I've maintained my vow.

But every night, while Brittany and Lil cuddle on the couch, I shower and wash off the smiley veneer. I am happy. But I am terrified. My world could change at any moment. The water hits my head, runs down my face, and washes down the drain. The showers heavy spray mutes my cries.

I towel off, dress, and lie with my two ladies. I crack a joke making them both laugh. The weapon is out.

HEMORRHAGE

The plan was simple. The high-risk delivery doctors, the oncologist, the anesthesiologist, the urological surgeon, all scheduled. They even reserved enough blood bags to transfuse a person three times. The date two weeks away, Brittany and I lie in bed and discuss the plan for having guests over. Our families want to help. But our home is tiny. It's a beach bungalow – two tight bedrooms and a single bathroom with a fitter tub that thumps if you stand in the wrong spot. I often wonder when it'll cave in and I'll smash through the tub floor and crash into the crawlspace below. "This house doesn't have space for a lot of company," says Brittany. My mind leaves the crawl space.

"We're not going to care where people sleep. That will be the last thing on our minds," I say, as I raise my voice.

"But it has to be normal for Lil. We can't change her world. It will be different enough with a sister. We have to keep things normal." She cries.

In my stubbornness, I realize what she's actually thinking about. She's been reading a few Facebook pages built for women with the same condition. The stories are horrible. One woman got transfused six times and wound up in a coma. Another woman passed away. Another went home fine and then hemorrhaged later at home and wound up back in the hospital. Brittany sees her fate and wants to protect our daughter from the looming trauma.

We roll over and close our eyes.

Later, I feel Brittany stir and get out of bed. She disappears into the bathroom. After a few minutes I wonder if the tub opened up and swallowed her. "Matt," she whispers. "Come here."

She's in the small hall space between our bedrooms and the bathroom, holding her stomach. "I'm bleeding. I have the doctors on the phone." She hangs up and wipes her tear-covered cheeks. "Time to go. They're heading in now. There goes the schedule. I texted my mom and she's on her way. She'll stay with Lil and be here when she wakes up."

The commotion wakes Lil anyway.

Her mom stands at our front door as Brittany shuffles around inside the house. "She'll be okay," says her mom.

"I know," I say and hug her. She's telling herself this – not me. Comforting herself that her oldest daughter will be coming home in a week.

As we leave, Brittany's mom sits on the couch and plays with Lil. We wave one last time. *She'll be okay*, I tell myself.

I DON'T WANT TO DIE

Brittany sits in a wheelchair outside of the OR as hordes of doctors and nurses flurry inside and out. They run back and forth, wearing their identity cloaking scrubs and paying little attention to us. Even our friend, the nurse on duty, is too busy to stop. Tears run down Brittany's face and she stares past everyone, past me.

A taller woman approaches Brittany and pulls down her mask. "Are you comfortable, hunny? What can I get you?"

"I'm cold," says Brittany. Which makes sense. The OR is balmy and Brittany wears nothing but her paper gown.

"Get this girl a blanket," yells the woman. "Let's take good care of her."

Someone runs over with a blanket. "I'm your anesthesiologist," she says. "What else?" She wraps Brittany and rubs her back.

Brittany's eyes drip redness. "I don't want to die," she says.

"Oh, hunny, you have the A-team here this morning. You're going to get your surgery. You're going to have your daughter. Tomorrow, you'll be recovering. And all this will be a memory." She rubs Brittany's back more, almost hugging her. "You're not going to die." She looks right at Brittany. "Okay?"

"Okay," says Brittany.

She peers at me. "Okay, Dad?"

"Okay," I say.

Some of the fear dissipates from Brittany's face. I squeeze her hand. We both needed that directness. "You'll be fine," I say. "It's the A-team."

Who is the hell is the B-team?

SHE'S A WHOPPER

Doctors and nurses filled the OR when Lil was born. There seemed to be two dozen. Now, because of Brittany's accreta, an army of doctors and nurses flood the room. They're after two goals – deliver the baby and keep Brittany alive. How hard can it be?

Once more Brittany disappears into the packed OR and I sit out in the long, green hall. Alone and quiet except for the faint beeping coming from behind the heavy OR door.

My whole life, everything I care about and love, now in the hands of a medical army. For weeks, we've only imagined this situation. Now, the cutters and sewers and saviors are in action. They hope not to lose her. I hope they can save her. They act. I watch.

They call me in.

"Sit behind the screen," says the anesthesiologist. Brittany looks confused. She's aware of the situation yet off somewhere else, the medicine working. I sit next to her head, find her hand, and squeeze it.

"You're doing great," I say. "Soon this will all be over." This whole situation will be over, but I have no idea how it will end. I am terrified. Hopefully she survives and the baby survives and we go home. In the best scenario, she will go home empty, a slice in her belly and a void in her abdomen – a reminder of her ruined dreams.

The room quiets down and the main doctors, two brothers, talk. "Everyone, you know your jobs. Communicate. Think quickly. Brittany and Matt, you're in great hands. Everyone ready?"

"Yes."

"Here we go."

In a blink everyone scurries around the two doctors as they lean over Brittany's stomach, handing them tools and rags. They talk and shout behind the screen that shields our view. One of them pokes his head up and toward us. "Brittany, let me know if you feel any pain. You might feel pressure, but not pain." Then he calls across the room. "Make sure we have that blood ready."

The anesthesiologist leans over Brittany's head. "I'll make sure you don't feel a single pinch of pain, dear."

"Thank you," I say. She smiles behind her green mask and her eyes scrunch up. "Of course, dears."

A minute goes by. The doctors speak a language we barely understand. "She's out," one of them says.

The team of NICU doctors pulls Lainey from his hands and Lainey yelps in raspy baby cry.

They carry Lainey to the incubator and tray table. They begin their initial checks – her weight, height, breathing – all the most important things. “She’s four pounds,” says a nurse.

“What?” I look at Brittany. “You hear that? Four pounds. She’s enormous. She’s a whopper compared to Lil. Will she even fit in Lil’s clothes?”

Brittany smiles at me. “Is she okay?”

I turn to the NICU team. “Her vitals are okay. We’re taking her up to the NICU now. You can come up with us and then come back down to check on Brittany,” they say.

Before they do, they wrap Lainey and lay her next to Brittany’s face and we smile for a picture.

I stand and kiss Brittany’s forehead. “I’ll be right back.”

“Kiss her for me if you can,” she says.

I'M AN ANESIESIOLOGIST

The NICU doctors assure me Lainey is doing fine. So I dash back to the OR. Fully scrubbed in, I stand next to Brittany and freeze. Her midsection is splayed open like an oversized duffle bag. Organs stretch over her sides and outside of her body. I'm not sure if I walked back in on a surgery or a scene from a horror movie. Regardless, I can't look away.

The doctors talk. "Her cervix needs to be capped. No space," says one doctor. "Here, I'll hold this down and you get it tight."

None of this bothers me – the organs, the blood, the butterfly filleted stomach. It amazes me. I watch with a clear view of it all. A doctor looks at Brittany, his hands fully stuffed inside her open stomach cavity. "Do you feel pressure, Brittany?" he asks.

"No."

"What's her level? We're putting her back together and I don't want her feeling anything."

The doctor stares at me.

"What's her level?"

I stare back. "I have no clue."

"Holy shit. You're standing there like that and I

thought you were the anesthesiologist."

"No, but I did stay at a Holiday Inn Express last night," I say.

Laughter fills the room. The anesthesiologist puts both hands on my shoulders. "Look back over here," she says. "We watch those numbers, with the green, glowing background. And they're fine."

"Thanks," says the doctor.

"He didn't pass out when he first came back in, so I figured he'd be okay to watch. It's kind of impressive," she says.

"It's amazing to see," I say.

The moment is over. The doctors and nurses and specialists go heads-down to save her life.

COUNT 'EM

"Okay," says the doctor. "I'm about to close her up. Let's do our count." He looks at the head nurse. "How many forceps?"

"Five."

"How many do we have?"

Another doctor gathers the used forceps and counts them out loud. "Three, four, five. Five. We're good."

"Knives?" asks the doctor.

"Eight," says the nurse.

"Five, six, seven, and eight," says someone else. The knives clang as the nurse drops them onto a metallic pan.

"Rags?"

"What are they doing?" I ask.

"Making sure we don't send your wife home with a rag stuffed in her belly," says the anesthesiologist.

"Twenty rags," says the nurse.

"Count them all," says the doctor.

"Twenty," someone calls out. "They're all here."

"Good. Okay, closing her up."

WE GOT THIS N.I.C.U THING

The maternity ward is completely changed. It's updated and comfortable and resembles a hotel room. And it seems closer to the Level Three NICU, where we'll be with Lainey.

"Like the renovations?" asks a nurse as she walks into the room. "We think it'll be better emotionally for the mom and the baby. But you're the first guests, so you'll have to let us know."

Brittany hugs the familiar nurse. "Hi, Guerly," says Brittany.

"I'm Lainey's nurse," says Guerly.

It's a relief. She had a few shifts with Lil and was fantastic. Her humor made the crappy more happy. Hopefully she'll do the same as Lainey's head nurse.

Brittany lies in her bed. We've got this. We've been here before and this is nothing different. It will be tough with Lil at home, but we know the drill. Lots of alarms, lots of worry. But we'll be fine.

"You're thinking," says Brittany.

"I am. In a way, I'm glad we've been down this road. We've been here before. It sucked. But we can do this again."

“Nothing’s ever exactly the same in here,” says Guerly. “It’s never routine.”

“Got it,” I say. “Still though. We know the drill.”

PARENTS TO THE RESPITE

Before Brittany left the house for the hospital – hemorrhaging – we had been arguing over who would come stay with us after she delivered. Brittany and I are different. She's mostly an introvert. And I am mostly an extrovert. She's happy with having a single friend over for Christmas dinner. I'm happy having the entire neighborhood over for Christmas dinner. Brittany wanted her Mom around. I wanted everyone and her mother over.

She dug in her heels. I dug in mine. We went to sleep. A couple hours later she was crying and bleeding in the bathroom. Our thoughts changed from *who will stay over at the house* to *I pray Brittany survives this and comes home.*

My parents, Lil, and I walk the boardwalk on the beach in Point Pleasant. A few of the rides are open for some reason and a few of the small shops are open. Lil runs around with us, oblivious to the trauma that's unfolded. For her, life is as sunny as the day and as exciting as taking a ride on the spinning teacups.

The air is crisp and the sun warms my face, and as we walk the boards and chat and chase Lil, for that moment, life is good.

We snap a picture, my parents and Lil sitting on a bench overlooking the rollercoaster and the little motorcycles, everyone smiling.

After a couple of exhaustingly fun hours, we walk back to the car. Lil is passed out, sleeping in my arms with her head on my shoulder and her drool dripping down my back. I snuggle her tight. “I’m here,” I say. “I’ll always be here.”

We settle in the car and head home and I breathe deep and look at my dad in the passenger seat and at my mom in the back with Lil. “Thank you,” I say. “Thank you.”

2AM CODE RED

I don't sleep on a normal night. My body doesn't need it. Closing my eyes at 2am and waking at 5am is routine. Tonight is different. I'm home with Lil. We didn't want her routine to be too extraordinary.

I'm exhausted, having pulled all-nighters for a few days and unable to rest. Tossing and turning on the couch, I pull the covers over my head. The blanket provides just enough solace that my eyes droop.

My phone buzzes. "Hi," I say.

"She's not okay." It's Brittany.

"What?"

"Lainey. She's not breathing on her own. The doctors said she's coding." Brittany strains giving me the information through her sobbing. "This was supposed to be easier. She's older. She's heavier. Why is this happening?"

"Because she's already being a brat and she's punished," I say.

Brittany laughs a little. "I'm so scared. They're hooking her up to a breathing machine now."

What should I do? My wife and my baby are 20 minutes away and need me. But my other baby, my

Lil, is home. If she wakes up and I'm gone, she'll know something is wrong. She loves her grandmom but waking up to her and not her dad the first morning back is far from normal routine.

"What do you want me to do?" I ask Brittany. "Because I have no idea what the right answer is here."

"I don't know," she says. "If you come here, you're leaving Lil. If you stay there, I'm dealing with this on my own. My mom is here. She could switch with you. But I don't know what the right answer is."

"What is the doctor saying?"

"That she's not in good shape. But they're doing everything they can to get her breathing."

"We have to keep things normal for Lil, too. Do you think I have to be there?"

"No. If it comes to that, I'll call you."

"You're sure?"

"No."

Neither am I. Once again forced to choose between being with my wife and Lainey and being with Lil. Who the hell is pulling the strings?

"Okay, I'll stay home. Call me if it gets worse and I'll get there as fast as possible. But call me and update me."

We hang up and I walk into Lil's room. She's sleeping on her belly, her breathing calm. I sit on the rocker next to her bed and watch her until she stirs and wakes for breakfast. No phone calls and no texts with updates. Lil smiles and laughs seeing me. "Daddy!"

I pick her up and we start her routine.

TINY SLICE

Both lungs collapsed. But after a tube and some panic, she's breathing. The tiny slice under her armpit barely bleeds and the tube is the thickness of a toothpick. It hangs out of her torso and blends in with all the other cords and hoses that drape from her preemie body.

I pull my index finger from inside her hand and touch her new wound. Less than a quarter of an inch. Her doctor's ability to cut less than a quarter of an inch saved her life. I slide my fingertip from her wound to her chest and I gently rest my palm across her heart. Her little bursting breaths push my hand up and down.

My eyes close. "I'm so sorry, Lainey Kate."

I cry until Brittany wakes up.

FIVE-DAY WAIT

Brittany and I sit in a closed-off room in the NICU. My yellow paper robe flows freely from my body as I pace back and forth from the window to the door.

"What?" asks Brittany.

"I'm excited," I say.

Brittany just smiles at me. I'm a terrible poker player.

Lainey was born five days ago. Today we get to hold her for the first time. Yes, we'd been through this with Lil. Yes, this wait should have been easier. But I can't wait to cradle her teeny body in my forearms and whisper in her ear that I'll never let anything bad happen to her.

The poor four-pound lass had already gone through so much – early birth, collapsed lung, feeding tubes – and I could never just scoop her up and make it okay.

Guerly walks into the room and sees us both beaming. "Little excited," she says.

"Yup," says Brittany. "Hard to tell, I know."

"Well, Mom holds her first."

Brittany readies herself and sits in the comfy

reclining chair and pats down her gown and fixes her mask. She's ready and I can see her nose crinkle behind her mask. The thin protective paper can keep germs in and out but it can't contain Brittany's happiness.

Guerly opens the incubator, sliding some of Lainey's cords around her elbow. She gently picks up Lainey and guides her four-pound body and 10-feet of cords and tubes over to Brittany's waiting arms. "I'll leave you three alone. I'm right outside if you need anything," says Guerly.

"I love you," I say to Brittany.

"I love you, too."

Once again, our first time holding our child is vastly different than others. We waited five days. Lainey is hooked up to a wall of machines and computers, cords dangling from her like Frankenstein's monster. Brittany and I are covered in protective gear like we're battling an Ebola outbreak, unwilling to even lower our masks in fear of spreading germs.

But it's our moment. Different? Yes. No less joyous. In some ways, maybe we'll remember this just like we remember our first time holding Lil. Brittany kisses Lainey's forehead through the mask and I see tears running down Brittany's cheeks.

It's beautiful.

Now hurry up so I can hold her!

BRITTANY'S SCAR

Brittany spends her time in her bed either holding Lainey or resting, still in pain from her surgery. With all the stress of Lainey's lungs collapsing, I've forgotten about Brittany.

She's sleeping. She looks content but wounded. I run my finger down her hairline.

"You're not out of the woods, yet, but I know you're not worried about yourself," I say, without waking her.

And it's true. Selflessness. Unchecked selflessness. Since having Lil, Brittany has spent very little time on herself. And as much as I promise her that I will make time so that she can get that hour or two a day to just go do something she wants to do, we find it difficult – I'm on the road. When I am home and I offer to give her time, she always responds selflessly. "When you're home, we should all spend time together." She's beautifully impossible.

She lies quiet and recovering. She won't show worry. But I do worry. As we had read when she was first diagnosed with accreta, there are risks during delivery – the woman can bleed out. But there are risks after surgery. Most often, the woman leaves the hospital and believes she's in the clear. But she's not well internally. The hysterectomy too much, she bleeds out a few days later.

"Don't you fucking dare," I say to her. Lainey sleeps quietly in her incubator next to Brittany's bed. Her alarms are silent, her breathing calm. "The two of you," I say, "you're both coming home."

I say it and half believe it. I know that coming home will be miraculous. I also know that Brittany's scar will forever remind her of what she went through and of what she can't have. It's a four-inch line of skin. It was the choice between a healthy baby, her own life, and the future of our family. "I'm so sorry," I say. "You're even more selfless than me when you're sleeping."

WHO NEEDS SKIN?

Lil roared into the world in March. Late March. Spring had sprung. Flu season had ended. In the NICU, we washed our hands and donned our paper scrubs and masks, always protecting the babies. But Lainey was born in November – the beginning of flu season.

I dig the harsh soap into the skin on my hands. Steam bellows from the sink and covers my face. Scrubbing up to my elbows, I count to 60 and then flick off the water, dry my hands, and head in to see Lainey.

Later that night, I scrub in again. Some soap – it seems – is intended to coax germs from our hands. This soap is intended to destroy any possibility of germs. Instead of foamy and fun scented, the soap is gritty and smells like fresh squeezed orange juice. I rub it into my hands and forearms. I hear Guerly's warning over and over … "These babies cannot get the flu. Lainey cannot get the flu."

Day after day, I massage the coarse germ killer into my skin. Day after day, my skin destabilizes. After two weeks, my hands crack and my knuckles bleed. It hurts to make a fist. It hurts to move my fingers. I can't even put my hands in my pockets.

I stand at the small pedestal sink outside the NICU doors with my mother-in-law. "My hands are so cracked," she says.

"I know. It's painful washing them. They bleed after they dry."

I count to 30, thinking it's sufficient, and grab a paper towel.

"How was your work trip this week?" she asks.

"Was good. The plane is always delayed," I say.

The plane. The filthy plane. A sign over the sink says, *It's flu season. Wash your hands and wear your mask.* "Ugh," I say. "I'll be right in." I load up more gritty skin and germ destroying soap and lather it onto my hands and forearms. And I count to 60.

EMPTY HANDED AGAIN

Brittany and I walk up our driveway. I have laundry bags slung over my shoulders and my arms cradle flower vases against my chest. Straining to keep it steady, I nod at Lil who stands behind our glass storm door, a smile stretched across her face. Brittany holds her handbag and her pillows. She's cry-smiling.

We're empty handed.

Other families get to return home together - baby and mom. Our family's not complete … once again. Not whole yet. Lil pushes open the door and hugs Brittany at the top of the steps. Brittany's alive. Lainey's alive. We may not be complete yet, but at least we'll have the chance. Don't fuck this up, Lainey – the first time I threaten my Lainey.

Lil's carefree giggles fill our bungalow. For a moment, we focus on the present. This is life until Lainey proves she's ready to come home.

THE SONGS WE SING

I walk through the NICU doors. It's the first night I'm back by myself. Brittany is home with Lil, wrapping her in love and attention, for which we'll have to share more evenly from now on. I still don't know how I'm going to do that. For now, I'm going to spend some time with Lainey, just the two of us.

I walk into her room. It's dark. The lights are off and only the green, dim bulbs on the machine illuminate Lainey in her incubator. "Hi, munchkin," I say.

With Lil, I realized there's nothing unusual about talking to a baby who's lying in a hotbox. They don't answer of course, but it feels more natural to chatter than it does to sit in silence. "I brought some books for us to read. But first, I figure we'll listen to some music."

Lil and I listened to Eric Clapton… and we still do. Just the other morning, we danced through the kitchen while blasting *They're Red Hot* on the Bluetooth speaker. But I've decided that Lainey and I should have our own set of songs.

I pull up a rolling chair and plop myself next to

her. She hasn't moved, but I don't care. We keep talking as I pull out my phone and open my music and thumb through my saved artists. *Avett Brothers* pops up first. "Avett Brothers?" I say to Lainey. "They have great music. Mommy and I saw them live when she was pregnant with you, actually. Let's listen to a few of these."

So I scroll to the album *Mignonette* and play the first song – *Swept Away.* It's acoustic and slow flowing. Folksy. And it's a love song about how a woman jumped into a man's life and swept him away. First song. First line. First chorus. It's perfect.

"This is our song, Lainey." I lean my forehead against her incubator glass. "You know you've already put us through hell. But you're ours. And you're a fighter. And Mommy and I are here for you to fight with you. And we will be forever. And so will Lil. You're going to love her."

The song ends with the chorus *And you… swept me away.* "You really have swept me away, Lainey."

She sleeps, not noticing the music or my banter. I cross my arms on the incubator and rest my head and cry.

SIBLING VISITS

Diana visits. I check her in and then we sit with Brittany and Lainey. "Lainey, this is your Aunt Diana. She's my older sister." Diana hugs me and wraps me in her arms, protecting her little brother.

Maria visits. I check her in and then we head to the NICU. "Lainey this is your Aunt Maria," I say. "She's my little sister, just like you're Lil's little sister."

Maria presses her hand against Lainey's incubator and then she folds her head down into my shoulder, just under my chin, and I hug her. "I'm okay, sister. We're okay." I cry through my mask.

Raymond visits. We stand over Lainey's incubator. "Lainey, your Uncle Stinky is here. He's my younger brother. Yes, he's taller than me," I say.

"She's so cute," says Raymond.

"She's put us through hell already. Going to be a wild one. I can tell."

Raymond lays his arm around my back and puts his hand on my shoulder and hugs me. "She'll be fine," he says.

"She will be," I say, and cry through my mask.

DIRTY PETER RABBIT

Lainey and I take advantage of late-night visits. With work done and Brittany and Lil home, I make the 20-minute drive to the NICU around 10pm. It's our time. The setup is simple. We listen to some Avett Brothers on my phone and I read her books.

Tonight, I've brought over the entire Peter Rabbit boxed set. The plan is to read a few and just sit. We've been doing this almost every night. She lies there while I share my thoughts. It's a one-way relationship but I know she'll make up for it when she's older.

"Hi," I say. "Ready for the first book?" I pull the first thin, pink book out of the box. I've picked this series because, while I've heard of Peter Rabbit, I've never read the books. Never even heard of most of the characters.

I'm a few books in and I switch the music to Grateful Dead. We're relaxed. It's almost time to change Lainey's diaper. So I sit with the next book. The cover has a cat on it and the background is a light purple. I'm on page two and this children's series takes an unexpected turn – "The pussy –" What the hell is this? It's a kid's book. I read a few more pages and there it is again – Pussy. Of course it means cat. Beatrix Potter meant no harm in using the word pussy. Back when she wrote this, the word pussy wasn't used the same way. The author probably never envisioned my situation – a father reading to his daughter and laughing when he hits the word pussy. The author didn't think about her reader's maturity level. She should have.

I should have realized that the series and its lessons are dated. The first book is about Peter, who gets his ass blown off by the farmer's shotgun. I chuckle and Lainey stirs. "We'll keep going," I say. We finish the pussy book. It's touch-time, so I put the boxed set under Lainey's incubator and open the lid. "Tomorrow we'll read something less dirty," I say. She grunts and rolls over. "Okay, okay, whatever you want is fine."

LIL MEET LAINEY

Today's the big day. Sisters meet for the first time. But it feels more like I have Lil at a baseball game and we're ordering food at the concession window.

"She has to stay behind the glass," says Guerly. Lainey, doing much better, is on a lower level of the NICU. It's less fancy and individualized – a room with incubators. Chiming heart and lung monitors ring day and night. Lainey sleeps soundly.

We drive to the hospital, Lil buckled in the back in her car seat next to the empty car seat. Soon they'll be sitting back there together, talking to each other. They'll laugh between phrases of kid blabber. Brittany and I will laugh at their laughter but have no idea what they're saying.

That beautiful bond starts today. "Lil," Brittany says, "one of us will stay with you. And one of us will go and hold her up to the glass so you can see her. But you won't be able to touch her or go in."

"Kay," says Lil.

"And she's not coming home with us," says Brittany.

"Kay," says Lil.

We arrive at the hospital. Lil skips down the hall, prancing with excitement. "Will she say hi?"

"Not yet," I say. "She's too little."

"Kay."

We get to the plexiglass that separates the NICU from the exterior hall. Lil stands on a chair and presses her forehead against the glass. I put my arm around her back and brace her. Embrace her. I could push her from the chair and onto the floor, but she'd still have that smile stuck to her face. This is the best day of her life that she won't remember.

Thousands of days of worry lie ahead for me. Today is my first day of completeness. Secret tearful nights and chest squeezing stressful days wash away. We're all together, even if separated by this two-inch pane of glass.

Brittany taps the glass and I smile. She holds Lainey up high, cradled in her arms and swaddled in her blanket. Only a few wires poke out. Brittany holds Lainey's hand up and waves it at Lil.

"She's waving, Dad, she's saying hi. Hi, baby," Lil says.

Brittany's chest heaves as happy tears run down her face. This is the best day of her life that she will remember.

LATE-NIGHT STOPS AT THE INLET

Nights are quiet. The graveyard staff works the NICU and the babies sleep. I hold Lainey against my chest, the lights dim overhead. We rock in a chair and talk about the day's events. I tell her Mom's report from that afternoon – Lainey's bells rang a few times because her heart rate raced. And she pooped twice. I tell her about work and how those with no passion for their jobs – coasters – bother me. "There are no coasters working the NICU," I say, "you little buggers keep them too busy."

Each night, we sit together from 10pm until midnight. I change her diaper, kiss her goodnight, and head out. I drive home through the darkness with the music off and recharge my brain. The roads are as empty as the hospital. Everyone's gone to sleep and tucked in their worries.

Every night I drive down 35 south, park under the bridge, and walk to the edge of the inlet. The treacherous waters are calm at the top of the inlet, closer to the river. Here, the waterways spider off and fill various marshes. Leaning on a railing, I watch as a white egret peers into the water, its skinny legs puncturing the water's surface.

"I'm going to drive my life," I say to the egret. "I will control the decisions that I have to make. We had no control over having two preemies. But I won't roll over." The egret lifts a lean leg and walks closer to me. "I'm in control."

When I get home, Brittany's sleeping on the couch and Lil's sleeping in her room. Lil's white noise machine fills our bungalow, puts me into a trance and forces my eyelids shut. It's 3am I call the NICU. "I'm checking on Lainey," I say. This is the only control I have right now.

DON'T ARGUE STATISTICAL SIGNIFICANCE WITH ME

"I don't want Lainey leaving here hooked up to that damn monitor," says Brittany as we leave the NICU. We climb into our truck and Brittany eases herself onto the seat, wincing from the surgical pain. "I'm serious," she says.

Lil came home hooked up to a contraption that tracked her vitals and alarmed when they dipped or spiked. Sensors taped to her chest and feet. They easily unhooked. The alarms rang often and for no reason. To us the device alarmed because it was defective and not because Lil was defective. Looking back, it was a bullshit machine. At the time, as nervous new parents, there were no other options. We thought we wouldn't be able to sleep if it wasn't hooked up, no matter how unreliable.

"Lainey's been through enough. We've been through enough. If her vitals are a concern, they should have been a concern since she coded on day three. If we have to, we can get one of the less intrusive PulseOx. We deserve some normalcy."

And that's just it. Two premature babies. Two

high-risk pregnancies. A hysterectomy. Our family plans ripped from us. Our baby should come home without looking like Frankenstein's monster. Tears run down Brittany's cheeks. "I want normal," she says.

We head back to the NICU the next morning – the doctors want to review the discharge testing. We're tired, but I know we're getting close to normal. Whatever that is.

"They'll hook her up to extra equipment for 12 hours," says the head doctor. "The results will determine if Lainey goes home with a monitor."

"Why would she?" I ask.

"The data will tell us. She could have a hard time breathing or her heart could be stopping."

"She's been hooked up to your monitors 24-hours a day for three weeks straight. Wouldn't we know if her heart is stopping?" I'm challenging her and peeking at Brittany to see if she notices.

"Let's see the results," says the doctor in her pretentious sounding Russian accent. She walks away.

It's bullshit. It stinks of a backroom deal between the hospital and the monitor manufacturer. Make sure babies go home with the machines. They shake hands. Insurance pays. Damn the parents and their sanity.

I kiss Lainey goodnight. Her extra cords flow out of her crib. It's as if a squid has jumped in with her and its tentacles dangle over the edge. "You can do this, Lainey Kate," I say, and leave.

We stand in front of the Russian doctor. "Lainey stopped breathing three times last night. So, we're recommending she go home with the monitor," she says to me and Brittany. Brittany walks away down the hall. "I'll be in the car," she says as she disappears.

"Three times?"

"Yes, three times."

"No one called us. If her breathing stopped three times, someone should have called us."

"This happens all the time. We don't call parents every time an alarm rings." She walks away from me a bit. But I move closer.

"When we got here, we asked how she was through the night. And I called at 2am like I always do. No one said anything about her breathing stopping."

"Well – "

"We've been in here every day for hours at a time. Her breathing hasn't stopped once. If you had said that her breathing sped up too much, I'd have believed that." I challenge her and now she's either going to retreat or defend herself.

"Mr. DeVirgiliis, this monitor tracks more – " She rattles off doctor jargon in an attempt to outsmart me. "And statistically speaking – " Now I have her. My job revolves around data analysis.

"You've monitored her for three straight weeks and not once has this type of episode ever come up," I say as I cut her off. "All of a sudden you hook her up to another device and her breathing stops three times. Either your machine's shit or theirs is shit. So which is it? And don't fucking argue statistical significance or hide behind doctor-speak bullshit with me. I'm a consultant. I use big words and numbers to bullshit people all the time."

We stand in the middle of the hall outside the NICU room. "I see," she says. "We recommend you go home with the monitor. But you can override our advice if you'd like. You have to sign a waiver. We can't be liable. I'll get you the paperwork."

The doctor turns and walks into an office, the door closing behind her. I breath deep as my heart rate races. Thank god I'm not hooked up to the damn device – my alarms would be screaming. A little fight for normal is worth it.

CHRISTMAS BREAKFAST WITH SANTA

"Should we go or no?" Brittany asks.

We have tickets to eat breakfast with Santa at a local restaurant – The Wharfside. The place is nice, sits right on the docks and looks out over the Manasquan Inlet.

"I don't know," I say. I find it's easier to defer some of these pressing decisions so that I'm not blamed when they wind up being the wrong decisions.

"You're no help," says Brittany. Lil giggles in the den. We're standing in our bedroom. Lainey's empty crib sits next to our bed. "It will be a good, fun thing to do with Lil before we bring home Lainey. Lil's world is going to change forever."

"She's going to love her sister," I say.

"Of course she will. But she'll be sharing us. Poor kid doesn't know what's coming."

We leave the bedroom and join Lil who's just running around playing with her toys and carrying her giraffe bink in her hand.

"Want to go eat with Santa?" says Brittany.

"Yay," says Lil.

"There's our decision," I say.

We dress in our fancy Christmas pants and dresses and sweaters and head out.

The breakfast is crowded. All the tables are in one large, all-glass room. Santa's throne sits in the corner. The food, mostly buffet, lines an adjoining room. Decorated Christmas trees and wreaths and holly are placed meticulously in every square inch of the space. It looks like Brittany decorated.

Brittany, Lil, and I sit at a table right against the windows. The water is calm and the sky is mostly white, like a blanket is covering us. The water reflects the docks and boats. I stare out.

"You okay?" asks Brittany.

"Yeah, this is nice."

"Lil's loving it."

Lil eats food from the table and points at Santa as he walks the room.

"Is it wrong?" I ask.

"What?"

"It's kind of like our last meal as this family, this trio. You made it. Lainey made it. We're going to be a quartet soon. But this is nice."

Brittany smiles to reassure me that I'm not a

complete jerk. "It is nice and yes it's okay to think that."

We eat until we're full and Lil sits on Santa's lap and we enjoy the rest of the morning, a trio preparing for our Lainey.

HOME

Brittany carries the car seat through our front door and into our little big house. "We're home," she says.

Lil bounces from her bedroom and greets us. "Hi," she says, "hi, sister."

The four of us huddle in front of the door, unable to make it any farther because a group hug is more important. Brittany unhooks Lainey – still teeny – from the carrier and leans down to Lil's height. We push into one another and I feel Lil's hand on my knee. "She's so cute," she says.

We move to the couch. Brittany lies Lainey Kate on a giant donut pillow. She looks like a doll. She looks perfect.

Lil follows her. She sits next to the enormous pillow and kisses Lainey's head. Then she turns to us smiling, her nose scrunched like her mom's. "She's my sister."

Brittany and I stand there and take it all in.

Life may have tried to deal us a shit hand. We fought back. Lainey is home and healthy. Brittany is alive. Lil has a mom and a sister. And for me? Perfection. Ponytails can wait.

AFTERTHOUGHTS

If you asked me, *what's the hardest part of being a parent?* I'd say it's being a parent. Yeah, the whole damn thing is hard. If you asked me, *what's the hardest part of being a NICU parent?* I'd say it's the waiting to be a parent. We couldn't feed our preemie daughters, couldn't hold them, couldn't squeeze them, couldn't bring them home. We had to learn how to do everything. How to read the monitors, how to re-attach the electrodes and cords, how to change preemie diapers.

Lil is now eight-years old and Laincy is almost six-years old. They build couch cushion castles and don princess dresses. They dig in the mud searching for worms. They chassé and plié in ballet class and through our house. They paint their nails and lather glitter makeup on themselves, on Brittany, and on me. And they bicker and talk back and get upset with each other and with us. They're little girls and they're mostly healthy and sometimes sick just like any other kids. Through the busyness of school and dance and play, you'd think I'd forget about all that happened. But every day I try to remember just how lucky I am.

Lil came home healthy.

Lainey came home healthy.

Brittany survived and came home healthy.

We are a happy, healthy quartet.

If you asked me, *what would you change about your experience as a girl dad, as a preemie girl dad?* I'd say … I'd change absolutely nothing.

ABOUT THE AUTHOR

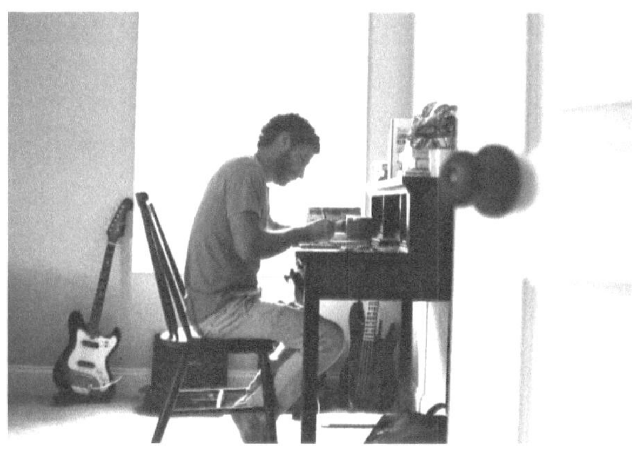

For Matt DeVirgiliis, the writing well sprang seventeen years ago and hasn't stopped.

He's written for the television networks Discovery Channel, TLC, HGTV, and BabyFirst Television. His short fiction and non-fiction have appeared in anthologies published by Pure Slush Books and Truth Serum Press; in *52/250 – A Year in Flash*; and in *Istanbul Literary Review.*

You can read most of his work at his website mattdevirgiliis.com.

Damn the Ponytail! is his first book.

THANKS

Thank you Brittany, Liliana, and Lainey for your supporting me and, at times, sitting with me while writing this.

And thank you, Peanut, for your uncanny speed-reading ability and willingness to critique.

Also from EVERYTIME PRESS

everytimepress.com/everytime-press-catalogue/

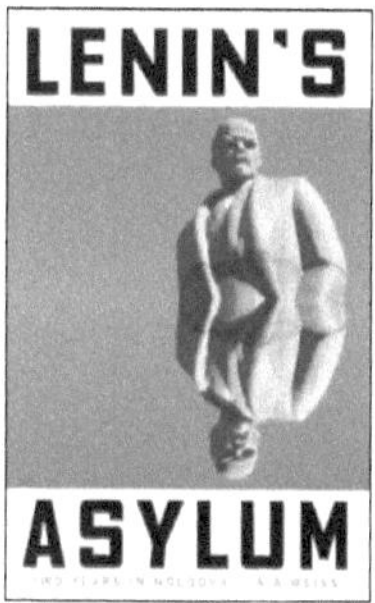

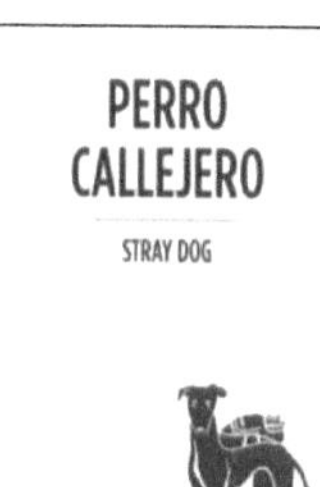

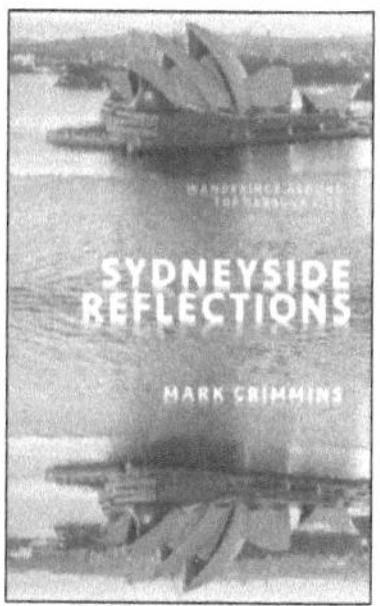

THIS IS ME,
BEING
BRAVE

PERSONAL ESSAYS

LEN KUNTZ

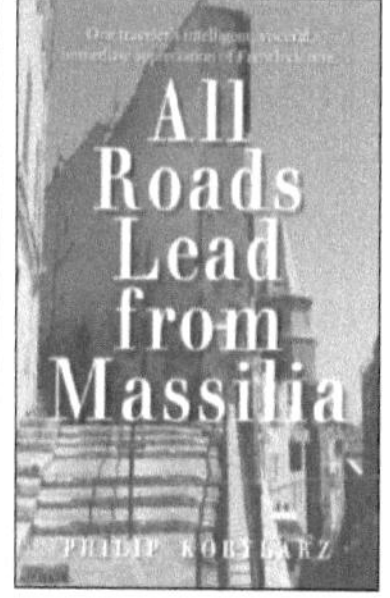

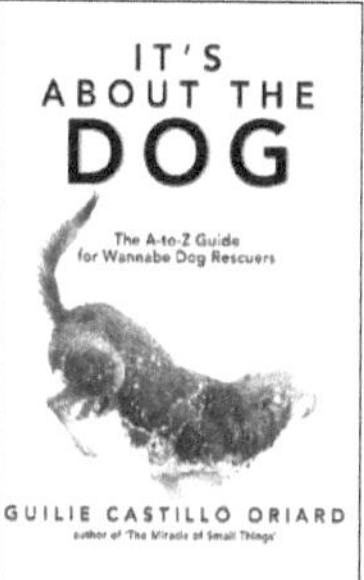

- Lenin's Asylum by A. A. Weiss
  ISBN: 978-1-925536-50-8 (paperback) / 978-1-925536-51-5 (eBook)
- Perro Callejero by Darren Howman
  ISBN: 978-1-925536-96-6 (paperback) / 978-1-925536-97-3 (eBook)
- Sydneyside Reflections by Mark Crimmins
  ISBN: 978-1-925536-07-2 (paperback) / 978-1-925536-08-9 (eBook)
- This Is Me, Being Brave by Len Kuntz
  ISBN: 978-1-922427-63-2 (paperback) / 978-1-922427-68-7 (eBook)
- All Roads Lead from Massilia by Philip Kobylarz
  ISBN: 978-1-925536-27-0 (paperback) / 978-1 925536-28-7 (eBook)
- It's About the Dog by Guilie Castillo Oriard
  ISBN: 978-1-925536-19-5 (paperback) / 978-1-925536-20-1 (eBook)